ACSM's Career and Business Guide for the Fitness Professional

NEAL I. PIRE, MA, FACSM

Owner, InsPIRE Training Systems
Ridgewood, New Jersey

 Wolters Kluwer | Lippincott Williams & Wilkins
Health
Philadelphia · Baltimore · New York · London
Buenos Aires · Hong Kong · Sydney · Tokyo

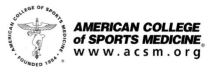 AMERICAN COLLEGE
of SPORTS MEDICINE
w w w . a c s m . o r g

Senior Publisher: Julie K. Stegman
Acquisitions Editor: Emily Lupash
Product Director: Eric Branger
Senior Product Manager: Heather A. Rybacki
Product Manager: Michael Marino
Marketing Manager: Christen Murphy
Manufacturing Coordinator: Margie Orzech-Zeranko
Designer: Karen Quigley
ACSM's Publications Committee Chair: Walter R. Thompson
ACSM's Group Publisher: Kerry O'Rourke
Compositor: SPi Global

Library of Congress Cataloging-in-Publication Data
Pire, Neal.
    ACSM's career and business guide for the fitness professional / Neal I. Pire. — 1st ed.
        p. cm.
    ISBN 978-1-60831-195-8
    1. Physical fitness—Vocational guidance—United States. 2. Physical education and training—Vocational guidance—United States. 3. Health—Vocational guidance—United States. 4. Personal trainers—Finance, Personal. 5. Physical fitness centers—Management. I. American College of Sports Medicine. II. Title.
    GV481.4.P57 2013
    613.7023—dc23

                                                                                2011028228

DISCLAIMER
Care has been taken to confirm the accuracy of the information present and to describe generally accepted practices. However, the authors, editors, and publisher are not responsible for errors or omissions or for any consequences from application of the information in this book and make no warranty, expressed or implied, with respect to the currency, completeness, or accuracy of the contents of the publication. Application of this information in a particular situation remains the professional responsibility of the practitioner; the clinical treatments described and recommended may not be considered absolute and universal recommendations.

The authors, editors, and publisher have exerted every effort to ensure that drug selection and dosage set forth in this text are in accordance with the current recommendations and practice at the time of publication. However, in view of ongoing research, changes in government regulations, and the constant flow of information relating to drug therapy and drug reactions, the reader is urged to check the package insert for each drug for any change in indications and dosage and for added warnings and precautions. This is particularly important when the recommended agent is a new or infrequently employed drug.

Some drugs and medical devices presented in this publication have Food and Drug Administration (FDA) clearance for limited use in restricted research settings. It is the responsibility of the health care provider to ascertain the FDA status of each drug or device planned for use in their clinical practice.

To purchase additional copies of this book, call our customer service department at (800) 638-3030 or fax orders to (301) 223-2320. International customers should call (301) 223-2300.

Visit Lippincott Williams & Wilkins on the Internet: http://www.lww.com. Lippincott Williams & Wilkins customer service representatives are available from 8:30 am to 6:00 pm, EST.

9 8 7 6 5 4 3 2 1

To Taryn and Nikki for their unconditional love
and never ending support. &

Preface

I was a chubby kid. I grew up in Brooklyn, New York, in modest surroundings, the only child of Cuban immigrants who had survived the depression, married, and came to the United States in search of a better life — ample opportunities of work, education, and food. My Dad was a laborer working long hours in New York City's garment district, and Mom, who spoke no English, was the primary caregiver at home. She made sure I was safe, by keeping me inside our one-bedroom apartment. She kept me "healthy" by making sure that I ate every last bit of food on my plate at each meal. She also made sure I availed myself to educational opportunities by providing books, drawing pads, arithmetic flash cards, and geographic jigsaw puzzles, which along with my "recreation" (a.k.a. television) kept me busy every minute of the day. Physical activity was work, and work was physical. Formal exercise was not part of my daily ritual, and its existence was well off my radar.

We later moved to Astoria, in Queens, New York, where I discovered "sandlot" baseball. Well, it was actually the demolition site of an elementary school, where the local kids gathered among the bricks and debris to live out their Major League dreams. Of course, the lot was eventually cleaned up for reconstruction, and we lost our ball-field, but no worries, there was always stickball, or strike-box, or manhunt, or stoopball, or anything else that a 12-year-old ingenuity could come up with to pass the time. Physical activity was all about playing games, and our games were physical. Exercising for its own sake was still unheard of in my corner of the world.

High school came along with a flurry of sports activities that were fun, competitive, and socially acceptable, if not expected. I also had the wonderful experience of a formal, comprehensive physical education program. Semester-long modules included gymnastics, basketball, speed-ball, team handball, and a host of other sports-related activities. It really opened my eyes to a whole new world of physical activity and sport. The physical fitness module was my first exposure to exercise for exercise's sake. I remember thinking that I was doing all of these exercises ONLY to become stronger and leaner. This was different from sports, because it did not provide the immediate gratification that scoring a goal or hitting a home run did. I felt as if I was doing it solely with the "hope" that I would become more fit.

It was during my teen years that I came across the old Charles Atlas ads in the back of comics, and of course, I didn't want any kid kicking sand in my face, so I ordered the Charles Atlas "Dynamic Tension" program. Wow! This guy came up with an exercise system that will buff me up fast. It didn't, and I dropped the regimen pretty quickly. Today I look back at it realizing that it was simply a total-body isometric exercise program, not the magic pill I had hoped for. Much like every other American adult, I wanted that easy fix. There was none!

I wrestled and played baseball in college, which required a regular workout schedule in addition to team practices, but all of the conditioning I was doing was still designed to enhance my performance not my waistline. As a result of all of my activity, however, I discovered that I could get in pretty good shape, but it required focused dedication over an extended period of time to get the significant results I was looking for. Upon hanging up my singlet, I decided that body-building was something I could do where I could apply my dedication, compete, and do something I had grown to enjoy — exercise. So off to the gym I went.

As an undergraduate student, I wanted to study biology and had an eye on premed. I got the opportunity to volunteer in the ER at Bellevue Hospital, famed for its gritty, fast-paced life-and-death environment. After one semester of gunshots and slashings, not to mention the nightly indigents suffering from gangrenous limbs barely hanging from their bodies, I came to my senses and decided I needed a more controlled clinical environment. I decided to volunteer in the physical therapy department at NYU Medical Center. This was great until 4 weeks into my tenure; I assisted my first neuro patient — a strapping, handsome 26-year-old motorcycle accident victim who was now in a semivegetative state. I was emotionally crippled! I wondered, "What can I do in health or medicine where I won't get so emotionally wrapped-up in my patient?"

A guidance counselor came up with recreational therapy. Mmmm...this sounds just right. So I signed on as a recreational therapy volunteer in the Pediatrics Department of NYU's University Hospital, where it seemed they flew the sickest kids from every corner of the world for treatment. I was assigned to a 10-year-old and would visit him twice a week to play games and help him pass the time. My 6th week in the program, I came to work, and my patient was no longer there. He had taken a turn for the worse and passed away overnight. I was blown away. Once again I was left wondering if there was any allied health field of study where I would not be dealing with such emotional situations.

That was when exercise physiology was brought to my attention. It was a field of study that allowed me to work with an "apparently healthy" population with the hopes of making them even healthier, more fit, and where applicable, improve their physical performance. I finally figured out what to study, but what would I do with my degree once I got out of school? Of those who stayed in the field, many graduates went on to grad school and teaching careers. Others embarked on careers in cardiac rehabilitation. There were others who worked at gyms and health clubs, teaching the general public how to exercise safely and effectively. This was a way to help people improve their health and performance doing something I personally loved doing. That was for me, and it is how my 30-year long career as a fitness professional began.

I share my personal story with you so that you understand what your journey may be or, perhaps, may have been. You might have a completely different experience, but it is likely that we shared some of the same fears and dreams along our career paths.

I write *ACSM's Career and Business Guide for the Fitness Professional* to serve as a guide and resource for the fitness professional, regardless of where you are in the continuum of your career. Ultimately, I want to feel, "If only I had a book like this when I was an undergraduate student...a rookie fitness instructor...a facility manager...a business owner/operator." This book is your "career guide" if you are interested in becoming a fitness professional or perhaps are already in the field, but you want to shift over to the "Management Tract." It will also provide a road map with valuable resources if you are a fitness professional and believe in your heart, "I can do it better" and wish to live out your entrepreneurial dreams. Read it and study it with an open mind and heart. Our field of "fitness" is still in its infancy, and dramatic growth lies ahead. Health clubs are a $20B industry and we know that their membership is comprised of only about 15% of the US population and, overall, only about 20% of the US population is physically active. What can you do to get to the remaining 80%? Good luck, and get to work!

Neal I. Pire, MA, CSCS, FACSM
Editor, *ACSM's Career and Business Guide for the Fitness Professional*

OVERVIEW – A USER'S GUIDE

The *ACSM's Career and Business Guide for the Fitness Professional* is intended to be a guide and resource for fitness professionals, regardless of their role in the industry or where they are in their career.

ORGANIZATION

This book is divided into three distinct parts.

Part 1 focuses on the fitness professional's career and his or her professional development. Chapter 1 identifies the more common "frontline" fitness professional careers, those of the fitness instructor, personal trainer, and group exercise instructor. It looks at professional preparation for these roles, identifying educational needs and professional credentials, with a comprehensive look at certification and accreditation, as well as licensure, which keeps popping up in proposed legislation in several states around the United States.

Chapter 2 describes the transition that many fitness professionals experience as they mature in their career and have to address a common "fork in the road": when the frontline practitioner decides to either continue to develop as a technician/clinician or expand his or her horizons and pursue a management or leadership role in the workplace. Chapter 2 also looks at fitness services as a value-added amenity of membership in a health club or fitness center and introduces common *a la carte* services that most commonly fall under the fee-for-service category.

Chapter 3 then presents actual sales strategies of fitness services, with a specific eye on selling personal training and selling health club memberships followed by some marketing and promotion, with a specific look at internal and external marketing, and most commonly utilized media in Chapter 4.

Chapters 5 through 7 focus on the delivery of the varied services and facility operations. They provide a general look at customer service models and risk management.

Part 2 includes Chapters 8 through 13 and focuses on the fitness professional as the entrepreneur. This part provides an overview of pertinent topics for starting and running a business — large or small — with some specific strategies and suggested resources where the budding fitness business owner can go for help. It outlines some basic rules of business plan and marketing plan writing, financial projections, and how to present a pro forma document to a potential investor when trying to secure capital for a business.

There is no entrepreneurial process more important than developing the business plan. The vast majority of small businesses fail within their first 2 years. Invariably those business owners never planned to fail. They just failed to plan. Part 2 is all about the creation, development, and selling of the business plan. It will take the entrepreneur through the process of clarifying the business' vision and developing every part of the business in a common sense, step-by-step manner leading ultimately to putting it all down on paper in the business plan.

Part 3 includes a complete sample business plan for a full-service fitness business featuring multiple programs with specific and unique target markets. This business project is to grow, opening four facilities during its first 5 years in business. This plan includes a marketing plan and, for the purposes of this book, only summary financials. A detailed financial plan should be included in any complete business plan, especially if the purpose of the plan is to raise capital to launch or finance part or all of the business. How to develop a detailed financial plan is described and outlined in Chapter 12 with start-up financials and marketing plan, as well as a sample presentation of the business plan that might be used when presenting the investment opportunity to prospective financiers. In addition, Part 3 also includes a sample operating budget for a different smaller business that demonstrates growth from its launch through its first 5 years in operation.

Note that at the end of each chapter readers will find "Your Resources" presenting easy-to-access information and business resources that have been highlighted within each chapter.

Acknowledgments

I wish to extend a heartfelt thank you to all of my professional colleagues who shared their thoughts and insights with me about the content and direction of this book. I would like to specifically acknowledge William Horne; his mentoring helped drive my desire to learn and develop my expertise of the business of fitness, so that I may share my insights here with other professionals and professionals-in-training.

On behalf of the ACSM and myself, I thank the many reviewers who volunteered their time and energy to ensure that the *ACSM's Career and Business Guide for the Fitness Professional* represents the current state of the industry and academia.

I thank the ACSM Committee on Certification and Registry Boards (chaired by Madeline Paternostro Bayles), the national staff of the ACSM Certification Department (Dick Cotton, National Director of Certification), and the ACSM Publications Committee (formerly chaired by Jeff Potteiger and now by Walt Thompson) for identifying the career and business aspects of the fitness profession as crucial to the success of today's professionals, important enough, in fact, to warrant the development of this book, and entrusting me to bring it to fruition.

I thank Kerry O'Rourke, ACSM's Director of Publishing, and our friends at Lippincott Williams & Wilkins, our publishing partners for this book. Specific thanks go out to Associate Product Manager, Michael Marino, as well as Acquisitions Editor, Emily Lupash, and Marketing Consultant, Christen Murphy, for their guidance and support throughout this project.

Finally, I thank the fitness professionals who touch and positively impact the health and lives of the masses, as well as to their managers, educators, and mentors without whom many careers would never flourish.

Contents

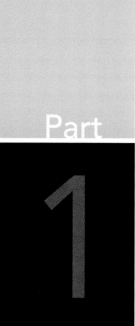

Part

1

The Fitness Professional's Career

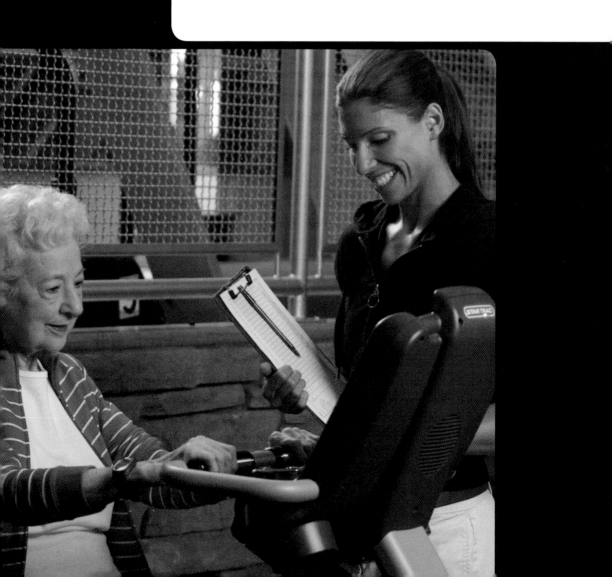

1 The History of a Profession

Chapter Objectives

After reading this chapter, the reader will:

- Understand a basic history of the fitness profession
- Understand the most general roles of fitness professionals in the fitness center or health club setting
- Understand the most common educational and professional credential requirements of fitness professionals
- Understand the basic purposes of credential and facility accreditation

FROM MUSCLE BEACH TO WALL STREET

The benefits of physical exercise for the mind, body, and soul have been touted throughout history. The great Roman orator, Cicero, was quoted, "It is exercise alone that supports the spirits, and keeps the mind in vigor." (2) Three hundred years earlier Plato expressed how detrimental inactivity can be, "Lack of activity destroys the good condition of every human being, while movement and methodical physical exercise save it and preserve it." (3) For centuries, it seems that we have always understood how important physical activity was to our well-being. Not until well after the industrial revolution, however, when daily routines became more automated and we were able to do so much more with so much less physical movement has exercise become a means and an end.

Some of us remember watching Jack LaLanne on television leading viewers through his signature circuit of calisthenics. It was a 30-minute show featuring a simple total-body progression of exercises highlighted by LaLanne's inspiring anecdotes and motivational stories. Who would have thought that nearly 60 years later there would be a cable television network devoted solely to teaching and motivating stay-at-home exercisers?

Jack LaLanne was one of the first mainstream fitness professionals to teach, lead, and motivate people to move and lead physically active lifestyles. There were others who came prior to LaLanne, but they were typically part of the "Physical Culture" movement and focused on unique specialties. Josef Pilates (1880–1967), for example, emphasized rehabilitative exercise that was intended for the unique benefit of dancers. Eugen Sandow (1867–1925), touted as the father of modern bodybuilding, was more a showman than an exercise leader or instructor. He did, however, popularize weightlifting, performing many signature feats of strength using a barbell.

As a publisher of many bodybuilding and fitness magazines, Joe Weider catalogued some traditional training methods, listing them as his own "Weider Training Principles." He also popularized bodybuilding as something that was beneficial and accessible to the masses. He brought Arnold Schwarzenegger from Austria and Franco Columbo from Italy to the United States and marketed them as part of the new California "body-beautiful" movement that had young kids running to their nearest Gold's Gym in droves to "pump iron."

The mom and pop bodybuilding gym evolved into what we might today call the "modern" health club. No longer a big room simply filled with barbells, dumbbells, and pulleys, today's health clubs feature an array of precisely engineered cardio and resistance training equipment that often requires thorough instruction on its basic operation, not to mention progressive planning to get the most out of its use. This need has historically been fulfilled by a fitness instructor.

Professional Roles — The Birth of a Profession

In the 1970s, the fitness instructor was someone who did everything in the health club: from spotting a lifter, to teaching a client how to use a treadmill, to providing a club member with a basic program card (often the only instruction available), to wiping down the mirrors in the facility. In the mid-1980s, the fitness instructor became a more specialized fitness professional. Clubs would often have personal trainers and group exercise instructors who specialized in individualized program design and instruction and group exercise leadership and instruction, respectively.

Today, the fitness worker, as the U.S. Department of Labor classifies the fitness professional, includes the personal trainer and group exercise instructor, as well as the fitness director, who typically oversees the fitness-related aspects of a health club (1). Each of these roles can be further categorized by training discipline or specialty, including yoga, Pilates, or strength and conditioning (typically providing sports performance–based training), among others. As these roles have evolved, so have their educational and training requirements.

Fitness Instructor

The role of the "fitness instructor" has evolved over the past 30 years. As gyms became "health clubs" and grew both in size and in scope of services, Mom and Pop operators had to provide some kind of supervision on the training floor. This role of the "floor trainer" was synonymous with what is more widely known as a fitness instructor. The fitness instructor's role often included anything and everything that needed to be done in the gym: from assisting exercising members, to spotting, to fixing and cleaning equipment. The fitness instructor was the fitness center's "jack-of-all-trades." Today, exercise programming and instruction is still often provided by the fitness instructor.

Personal Trainer

The personal trainer was one of the first "specialists" made popular in the industry during the mid-1980s. This specialist's primary role was to lead exercisers through their workout, educating and motivating them along the way.

The job required two core competencies including people skills and training skills. Personal trainers needed to have a passionate, engaging personality and an ability to "connect" with people, motivating them to exercise and push themselves well above their comfort levels to achieve new heights of fitness. They also needed to have knowledge and skills in exercise methodologies, in cardiovascular training and resistance training exercises, along with basic knowledge of anatomy and physiology, which became the "typical" toolbox for the personal trainer.

In the absence of formal educational or credential requirements, the typical personal trainer was an attractive, physically fit "gym rat" whose love for iron and the body beautiful oozed from his pores as it did passionately from his lips in every conversation he shared with anyone willing to listen. Clients often thought, "Wow! If I can train like him, I can look like him. I will hire him as my personal trainer." Looking the part was crucial then because there was no widely accepted standard for required knowledge and skill sets for the professional trainer. In other words, "If he looks good, he must know what he is doing."

Today, everyone wants a trainer who "walks the walk," truly believing in what he or she peddles on a daily basis. However, personal trainers' role and required toolkit have evolved into one that plays a more comprehensive role in clients' lives — one where personal trainers' understanding of a broad spectrum of knowledge is crucial to their ability to effectively help their client. In addition to basic exercise science, the well-equipped personal trainer's knowledge and skill set now include fitness assessment and program design, behavior modification and coaching strategies, the integration of recuperation strategies into a client's training program, and a basic yet broad understanding of some of the unique needs of certain clients who might have health- or performance-related limitations or requirements ("special populations").

This evolution has positioned the personal training profession as one that is poised for explosive growth over the next decade, while further evolving into a highly respectable profession and a rewarding career.

Group Exercise Instructor

The group exercise instructor has gotten a complete makeover, of sorts. Whether it was Jennifer Beals in *Flashdance* or Jamie Lee Curtis in *Perfect* that conjures up visions of torn sweatshirts hanging off your shoulder or bare feet and knit leg warmers, the group exercise instructor has evolved from performance artist to one of the toughest jobs in our industry — leading the masses in safe and effective exercise.

Adding to the innate challenges of the group exercise instructor's job, it is typically a part-time job with the instructor coming in to the facility, teaching the class and then leaving immediately thereafter. This presents a challenge for both the group exercise instructor and facility management. For the group exercise instructor, often an independent contractor, they do not have the same vantage point that the fitness instructor and other fulltime employees have. It is harder for them to get to know facility members, better understand their needs, and promote themselves and their classes. For management, they recruit and hire the group exercise instructor, investing at times even more time and money to do so than they do to secure their fulltime staff. In addition, it is challenging to manage this segment of your staff, because of its transient nature.

Fitness Director/Manager

A facility-based personal trainer may be hired or promoted to manage the personal training department, while still maintaining a schedule of training clients. This added responsibility requires good organizational and time management skills. Skills in interviewing, hiring, employee training, personnel management, record keeping, business management, risk management, health promotion, incentive programming, service pricing, marketing, sales, and policy setting will be needed by the personal training manager.

A fitness instructor or personal trainer may also be placed in charge of a fitness department in a health club, corporate fitness facility, or nonprofit recreational center. The personal trainers will probably be part of this department. In addition to overseeing the personal training sales and delivery, the fitness department manager may also be responsible for fitness equipment purchases, emergency drills, maintenance and repairs, special fitness programming events, and, in some cases, the group fitness program. Even with all of these responsibilities, the fitness manager may still be expected to retain personal training clients for additional department revenue and to supplement the trainer's salary received managing the fitness department.

Professional Preparation

The education and training required of fitness professionals depends on the specific type of fitness work. Professional certification has been the most widely used qualifier for personal trainers and group exercise instructors. An increasing number of employers require fitness professionals to have a Bachelor's degree in a field related to health or fitness, such as exercise science. Some employers allow workers to substitute a college degree for certification, but most employers who require a Bachelor's degree also require certification.

While requirements vary from employer to employer, most personal trainers must obtain certification in the fitness field to gain employment. Group fitness instructors do not necessarily need certification to begin working. The most important characteristic that an employer looks for in a new fitness instructor is the ability to plan and lead a class that is motivating and safe. However, most organizations encourage their group instructors to become certified over time, and many require it. In the fitness field, there are many organizations that offer certification.

Education

Certificate Programs

Many colleges, in particular community colleges, offer certificate programs in exercise science or adult fitness or a similar related field of study. These programs sometimes lead to an Associate's degree and can be part of the professional development of a fitness professional on the way to a Baccalaureate and more advanced degrees.

Degree programs

Degree programs vary in scope and depth but typically cover all of the pertinent coursework required by the frontline fitness professional. ACSM launched the

University Connection (UC) Endorsement Program (see Box 1.1), which was designed to recognize academic institutions with educational programs that cover all of the knowledge, skills, and abilities (KSAs) specified by the ACSM Committee on Certification and Registry Boards to prepare students for successful careers in the health and fitness and clinical exercise programming fields. The UC was phased out when the Commission on Accreditation of Allied Health Education Programs (CAAHEP) took over in 2010. CAAHEP has been providing a comprehensive "litmus test" for educational programs including those with a focus on personal fitness, exercise science, and exercise physiology. The Committee on Accreditation for the Exercise Sciences oversees these three programs and directly reports to CAAHEP.

BOX 1.1

ACSM UC Endorsement Program information is available at *http://www.acsm.org/Content/NavigationMenu/ Certification/UniversityConnectionEndorsementProgram/ UniversityConnectionEndorsedPrograms/University_Connectio.htm*

CAAHEP information is available at *http://www.caahep.org/*

Certification

Prerequisites

Prerequisites vary depending on the certification. Most accredited certifying bodies require a minimum age of 18 years, a high school diploma or equivalent, and current Cardiopulmonary Resuscitation–Automated External Defibrillation (CPR-AED) certification to qualify as a candidate to sit for the certification examination. All certification exams have a written component, and some also have a practical component or video component. The exams measure knowledge of human physiology, proper exercise techniques, assessment of client fitness levels, and development of appropriate exercise programs.

Some organizations offer more advanced certification, requiring an Associate's or Bachelor's degree in an exercise-related subject for individuals interested in training athletes, working with people who are injured or ill, or advising clients on general health and wellness coaching.

People planning fitness careers should be outgoing, excellent communicators, good at motivating people, and sensitive to the needs of others. Excellent health and physical fitness are important due to the physical nature of the job. Those who wish to be personal trainers in a large commercial fitness center should have strong sales skills. All personal trainers should have the personality and motivation to attract and retain clients.

Exam Preparation

There is no particular training program required for certifications; candidates may prepare however they prefer. Certifying organizations do offer study materials, including books, CD-ROMs, other audio and visual materials, and exam preparation workshops, seminars, and webinars, but exam candidates are not required to purchase materials to take exams. Certifying organizations have their own recommended list of exam preparation resources. ACSM offers a comprehensive Certification Resource Guide that helps examination candidates effectively navigate through the preparation process. It clearly defines and describes each of ACSM's five certifications, their scopes of practice, examination details, and a suggested list of resources to help prepare the candidate to sit for the examination. ACSM also offers online learning opportunities via its Learning Portal. Box 1.2 outlines some of the available examination preparation resources.

BOX 1.2   **EXAMINATION PREPARATION RESOURCES**

The current study kit for the ACSM Certified Personal Trainer^SM (CPT) includes

- *ACSM's Resources for the Personal Trainer*, 3rd edition
- *ACSM's Guidelines for Exercise Testing and Prescription*, 8th edition
- *ACSM's Certification Review*, 3rd edition

Additional online resources are available at the ACSM Online Learning Portal: *http://www.acsmlearning.org*

Live examination preparation workshops are also available. For more information, go to *http://www.acsm.org/Content/NavigationMenu/Certification/Workshops/ACSM_Workshops_Cer.htm*

Certification Renewals

Maintaining certifications typically requires documenting the successful completion of a prescribed number of approved or eligible Continuing Education Credits or Continuing Education Units, depending on the certifying organization. Credits are awarded based on contact hours completed in the given educational experience. Credits need to be earned during the term of the certification, which is usually 2 or 3 years, and some certifying organizations provide a grace period for certified professionals to document that they completed all of the requirements during their certified term and qualify for renewal.

Continuing Professional Education

There is what seems to be an endless variety of learning opportunities for the fitness professional. Many of these opportunities are delivered by preapproved

"CEC/CEU Providers," who have received approval from the certifying organization to provide the educational experience. Many certifying organizations also provide their certified professionals the opportunity to petition approval for specific educational experiences that had not been preapproved by their certifying organization.

Accreditation of Certifications

Professional certification affirms a basic level of proficiency for practitioners in a particular field. Certification represents a declaration of a particular individual's professional competence. An accredited certification is based on best practices and recognized processes and procedures developed by the field of certification.

National Commission for Certifying Agencies

Becoming certified by one of the top certification organizations is increasingly important. One way to ensure that a certifying organization is reputable is to see that it is accredited by the National Commission for Certifying Agencies (NCCA). Box 1.3 is a current list at the time of publication of NCCA-accredited fitness certifications.

BOX 1.3   **NATIONAL COMMISSION FOR CERTIFYING AGENCIES ACCREDITED CERTIFICATION PROGRAMS AS OF NOVEMBER 2010**

Dates listed below indicate that program's accreditation expiration date.

Academy of Applied Personal Training Education
- Certified Personal Fitness Trainer 3/31/14

ACSM
- ACSM Certified Personal Trainer^{SM} (CPT) 5/31/11
- ACSM Certified Clinical Exercise Specialist® (CES) 5/31/11
- ACSM Certified Health Fitness Specialist^{SM} (HFS) 5/31/11
- ACSM Registered Clinical Exercise Physiologist® (RCEP) 5/31/11

American Council on Exercise
- Advanced Health and Fitness Specialist 10/31/13
- Group Fitness Instructor 10/31/13
- Lifestyle and Weight Management Consultant 10/31/13
- Personal Trainer 10/31/13

The Cooper Institute
- Personal Trainer Certification 11/30/11

International Fitness Professionals Association
- Certified Personal Fitness Trainer 10/31/12

National Academy of Sports Medicine
- Certified Personal Trainer 4/30/11

National Council for Certified Personal Trainers
- Certified Personal Trainer 7/31/15

National Council on Strength and Fitness
- National Certified Personal Trainer 3/31/15

National Exercise and Sports Trainers Association
- Certified Personal Fitness Trainer 3/31/13

National Exercise Trainers Association
- Certified Personal Trainer 4/30/12
- Certified Group Exercise Instructor 4/30/12

National Federation of Professional Trainers
- Certified Personal Fitness Trainer 4/30/11

National Strength and Conditioning Association
- Certified Personal Trainer 10/31/13
- Certified Strength and Conditioning Specialist 10/31/13

Training and Wellness Certification Commission
- Advanced Certified Personal Trainer 3/31/14

Professional Licensure

The general purpose of licensure is public safety and ensuring the delivery of professional services. Licensure is typically mandated, governed, and administered at the State level. While there are no States currently requiring licensure for fitness professionals, there are several States that have introduced legislative bills that would require fitness professionals to acquire a license to practice personal training, group exercise leadership, and the delivery of other fitness services. While licensure would standardize the credentialing requirements for fitness professionals of a given State, it is important to note that such requirements may differ from State to State. As legislation is introduced, it is important for fitness professionals to be "in the know" and provide feedback to legislators from the profession's perspective.

Facility Accreditation

It is important to note that as the fitness profession has evolved, so has the industry. Validation in the consumer's eye and that of other professionals of both the fitness professional and the business entity or facility is important to its legitimacy and longevity. The industry is currently struggling to standardize its services across the board. A large and varied group of industry stakeholders have been working with NSF International, an independent, not-for-profit organization that certifies products and establishes standards in areas of public health to develop a fitness facility accreditation. The purpose of the accreditation is to establish criteria that raises the bar and ensures for fitness consumers and health and medical professionals alike that the facility's equipment, services, and staff meet standards that ensure quality and safety.

An important thing to note at the time of this publication is that staffing criteria are part of this industry initiative and that fitness professionals in training should heed to the proposed criteria, as they might be requirements for work at some point down the line. Box 1.4 outlines the current proposed staffing criteria in the facility accreditation document.

BOX 1.4

PROPOSED STAFF CREDENTIALING REQUIREMENTS IN NSF FACILITY ACCREDITATION DOCUMENT (AS OF MAY 2011)

Health/fitness professionals who have supervisory responsibility for the physical activity programs (*i.e.,* who supervise and oversee members and users, staff, and independent contractors) of the facility shall have an appropriate level of professional education, work experience, and/or certification. The examples of health/fitness professionals who serve in a supervisory role include the fitness director, group exercise director, aquatics director, and program director.

An aquatics director shall be compliant with the requirements mandated by local jurisdiction and have at least one of the following:

- Advanced Life Saving (ALS) or Water Safety Instructor (WSI) certification
- Minimum of 3 years' experience as a lifeguard, WSI, or swim instructor

In addition, facilities with pools shall have a staff person who has a recognized Certified Pool Operator (CPO) certification such as those issued by National Spa and Pool Institute or state/local government agency. This individual can be the aquatic director or other person charged with the physical care of the pool (pool chemistry and mechanical systems).

A fitness director must hold at least one of the following:

- Fitness Instructor or Personal Trainer certification, or its equivalent, from a nationally accredited certifying organization
- A 4-year degree from an accredited college or university in fitness, exercise science, or related field
- Have a minimum of 3 years' experience as a fitness professional in a health/fitness facility

A clinical fitness director must hold at least one of the following:

- A professional certification or license, or its equivalent, from a nationally accredited certifying organization
- A 4-year degree from an accredited college or university in fitness, exercise science, or related field, and have a minimum of 3 years' experience as a clinical fitness professional in a health and/or medical fitness facility

A group exercise director must hold at least one of the following:

- Group Exercise Instructor certification from a nationally accredited certifying organization
- Have a minimum of 3 years' experience as a group exercise instructor working in the fitness and health industry in a health/fitness facility

A program director must hold at least one of the following:

- A certification in fitness, group exercise, or related recreational field from a nationally accredited certifying organization
- Have a minimum of 3 years' experience working as an instructor or supervisor of physical activity or recreation programs

The health/fitness professionals who serve in counseling, instructional, and physical activity supervision and instruction roles for the facility shall have an appropriate level of professional education, work experience, and/or certification. The primary professional staff and independent contractors who serve in these roles are fitness instructors, group exercise instructors, lifestyle counselors, and personal trainers. Below are the criteria of what might be considered the appropriate blend of professional education, certification, and work experience for some of the relevant positions in the health and fitness industry.

A personal trainer or fitness instructor shall have a Fitness Instructor or Personal Trainer certification from a nationally accredited certifying organization.

A group exercise instructor shall have a Group Exercise Instructor certification from a nationally accredited certifying organization.

A lifestyle counselor, wellness coach, or its equivalent shall have at least one of the following:

- Certification from a nationally recognized certifying organization in lifestyle management, health/wellness coaching, behavioral change, or similar area
- Minimum of 1 year of experience working as a fitness instructor or personal trainer, with at least 100 hours' experience in lifestyle counseling or wellness coaching

Health/fitness professionals engaged in assessing or prescribing, instructing, monitoring, or supervising of physical activity programs for facility members and users shall have CPR-AED certification from an organization qualified to provide such certification. A certification should include a practical examination.

Advancement

A Bachelor's degree in exercise science, kinesiology (the study of muscles, especially the mechanics of human motion), or a related area, along with experience, is often required to advance to management positions in a health club or fitness center. Some organizations require a Master's degree. As in other occupations, managerial skills are also needed to advance to supervisory or managerial positions. College courses in management, business administration, accounting, and personnel management may be helpful, but many fitness companies have corporate universities in which they train employees for management positions.

Personal trainers may advance to head trainer, with responsibility for hiring and overseeing the personal training staff and for bringing in new personal training clients. Group fitness instructors may be promoted to group exercise director, responsible for hiring instructors and coordinating exercise classes.

Later, a worker might become the fitness director, who manages the fitness budget and staff. Workers might also become the general manager, whose main focus is the financial aspects of an organization, particularly setting and achieving sales goals; in a small fitness center, however, the general manager is usually involved with all aspects of running the facility. Some workers go into business for themselves and open their own fitness centers.

Fitness workers held about 235,000 jobs in 2006. Almost all personal trainers and group exercise instructors worked in physical fitness facilities, health clubs, and fitness centers. About 8% of fitness workers were self-employed; many of these were personal trainers, while others were group fitness instructors working on a contract basis with fitness centers. Many fitness jobs are part time, and many workers hold multiple jobs, teaching or doing personal training at several different fitness centers and at clients' homes (1).

CHAPTER SUMMARY

Chapter 1 described the rapid evolution of the fitness profession from a historical perspective. It outlined the primary roles of fitness workers: fitness instructor, personal trainer, group exercise instructor, and fitness director. It also provided an overview of professional preparation for a career as a fitness professional, including education and credentials, and provided background on the accreditation process for certifications and health fitness facilities.

YOUR RESOURCES

Professional Education Resources:
Commission on Accreditation of Allied Health Education Programs (CAAHEP)
http://www.caahep.org/

Committee on Accreditation for the Exercise Sciences (CoAES)
http://www.coaes.org/

Professional Credentialing Resources:
Institute for Credentialing Excellence — ICE (Formerly the National Organization for Competency Assurance) ICE is a nonprofit, 501(c)(3) organization dedicated to providing educational, networking, and advocacy resources for the credentialing community. ICE's accrediting body, the National Commission for Certifying Agencies (NCCA), evaluates certification organization for compliance with the NCCA *Standards for the Accreditation of Certification Programs. NCCA's Standards* exceed the requirements set forth by the American Psychological Association and the U.S. Equal Employment Opportunity Commission.
http://www.credentialingexcellence.org/

Facility Accreditation Resource:
NSF International — NSF International, The Public Health and Safety Company™, a not-for-profit, nongovernmental organization, is the world leader in standards development, product certification, education, and risk management for public health and safety.
http://www.nsf.org/

REFERENCES

1. Department of Labor, Bureau of Labor Statistics. *Occupational Outlook Handbook, 2008–09 Edition* [Internet]. Available from: http://www.bls.gov/oco/ocos296.htm
2. Hertzog C, Kramer AF, Wilson RS, Lindenberger U. Fit body, fit mind? Your workout makes you smarter. *Scientific American Mind, Scientific American* [Internet]. 2009 [cited 2009 July]; p. 24. Available from: http://www.scientificamerican.com/article.cfm?id=fit-body-fit-mind
3. National Plan for Physical Activity. [Internet]. 2008. Available from: http://www.physicalactivityplan.org/

2

A Fork in the Road: Technicians and Clinicians

Chapter Objectives

After reading this chapter, the reader will:

- Understand the most common fitness professional technical/clinical roles and their delineation
- Understand basic fitness facility service levels including common value-added services and fee-for-service options under a facility's profit center umbrella
- Identify the common compensation methods for each fitness professional role including that of the fitness professional who "wears many hats" and delivers services across the board

THE FITNESS PROFESSIONAL AS TECHNICIAN AND CLINICIAN

Many fitness professionals decide to embark on their fitness career because they have an innate vocation to help others. They want to be on the frontline, having direct and regular contact with the exercising public. For them, there is nothing more gratifying than helping someone achieve their fitness goals while making a tangible and significant positive impact on their health and longevity. This repeatable marker of success is why so many professionals passionately pursue a career in fitness with the acceptance and understanding that "they're not in it for the money." The primary role of all fitness professionals is to educate and motivate the public to participate in safe and effective goal-oriented exercise. The well-equipped fitness professional possesses all of the tools necessary to make such an impact.

It is important to note that there are fitness professionals who choose to prepare and serve as clinicians providing exercise as medicine or treatment for disease. The career paths for these clinical roles include formal education, requiring a minimum of a Bachelor's degree in Exercise Physiology, and more typically a Master's degree, along with clinical credentials such as ACSM's Clinical Exercise Specialist Certification or Registered Clinical Exercise Physiologist. For the purposes of this book, we will focus on the health-fitness professional, most often working in a health-fitness environment, not in a medical or clinical environment.

FITNESS AS A VALUE-ADDED SERVICE

Fitness instructors and group exercise instructors are typically the frontline professionals who are available to assist members in the health club or fitness center environment. Fitness instructors patrol the exercise floor wearing many hats, doing everything that needs to be done, and in some cases, even teach group exercise classes. Group exercise instructors are "specialists" who typically come in solely to teach a scheduled class. Some of the more traditional "gyms" do not have separate facilities where they can conduct classes, but many manage to run group cycling, circuit training, and other types of classes in designated areas right on the fitness center floor, as space and traffic allow.

In most fitness centers, services provided by fitness instructors and group exercise instructors are generally "value added," meaning that facility members do not pay additional fees for their services. Some facilities hire personal trainers to provide some basic fitness services (*i.e.*, fitness assessments, program design, etc.), where they have an opportunity to sell their personal training services to the member, converting them into a paying client. In most cases, this is a premium or "fee-for-service" ancillary service that requires the member to pay a fee above and beyond his or her membership dues.

Fitness instructors usually receive compensation based on an hourly rate of pay, which covers all services rendered with exception to fee-for-service training, for which they typically receive a premium above and beyond their regular hourly rate. Group exercise instructors usually receive an hourly or "class rate," which is a flat fee for each class they teach. They usually receive some kind of premium rate for any fee-for-service classes or training sessions they deliver in addition to their regularly scheduled classes. Personal trainers receive a "training rate" for every paid session they complete. In some facilities, personal trainers deliver complimentary sessions to new members, for which they will receive an hourly rate similar to that of the fitness instructor. In other cases, personal trainers do not receive compensation for these complimentary sessions. They deliver these sessions solely for the purpose of converting the member into a paying personal training client.

Service models differ widely from facility to facility, but most facilities provide some basic level of fitness programming inclusive with membership. It might be as simple as a program card with a basic resistance training circuit that the member can follow on his or her own or as comprehensive as a multiple appointment model with several facility personnel, including everything from preactivity screening and fitness assessment to hands-on training sessions following a customized training program designed specifically for the individual member. Figure 2-1 describes the new member flow in a service model commonly seen in many member-based fitness facilities.

Regardless of the model, all of these services may be delivered by a fitness instructor, depending on his or her professional experience and credentials, and the staffing model implemented at the given facility.

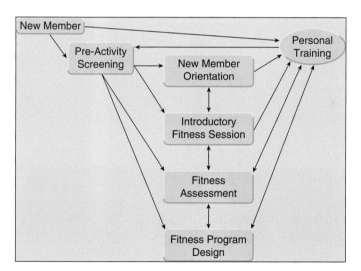

Figure 2-1. The diagram above describes various service models commonly seen in membership-based fitness facilities. New members enroll and are on their own from the get-go, which means they would pay for a personal trainer upon enrolling in order to receive assistance. The personal trainer would provide all exercise leadership, from preactivity screening, through program design and instruction. Alternative service models would provide some screening and introductory sessions that would ease new members' entry to the club, as part of their membership privileges. Personal trainers typically deliver these sessions providing opportunities to build rapport with new members and sell them the trainer's services. In both models, the ultimate goal is to sell new members personal training.

Fitness instructors are typically hourly or salaried employees who are compensated based on hours worked, and can receive additional commissions, bonuses or premium hourly rates based on the services provided. Group exercise instructors are usually hourly employees receiving compensation either by the hour or by the class. Both tend to fall under the value-added umbrella. The personal trainer, on the other hand, commands a premium pay rate derived from the fee paid by the client.

FITNESS AS A PROFIT CENTER

Personal training is the most common fee-for-service feature widely available across the board regardless of the size and type of facility (1). Personal trainers are often "hired guns," available to facility members for a fee, and receive a premium as part of their compensation. The compensation model depends on their work status or relationship with the facility, certifications, and education level. Some facilities' trainers are employees, others are independent contractors, and yet others are "solo" or independent business owners/operators who serve as vendors to the facility owner/manager.

The "solo trainer" is commonly known as a personal trainer who is independent of another business entity, most commonly their place of work. This trainer typically markets himself or herself to potential clients and schedules and delivers training sessions in the client's home, outside, or in the gym. The employee or independent contractor is typically hired or contracted by a business owner to provide training services for the business's clients. The personal trainer/manager/owner typically supervises all business operations and staff management of a personal training business (Fig. 2-2).

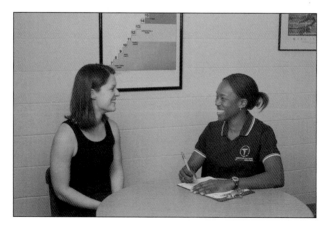

Figure 2-2. Personal trainer and her client communicating effectively. Reprinted with permission from ACSM's Resources for the Personal Trainer. 2nd ed. Philadelphia (PA): Lippincott Williams & Wilkins, 2007.

While the emphases on specific job tasks might differ from one setting to another, the goal is ultimately the same — to follow sound business practices and develop a profitable enterprise by delivering the optimal level of service to the end user, the training client.

There are various common compensation models for personal training programs in the fitness center setting. Some facilities pay trainers a percentage of the revenue generated by the services they deliver. Other facilities hire personal trainers as hourly or salaried employees with designated work shifts and pay the trainers an additional commission for "fee-for-service" sessions delivered to the members. Others hire personal trainers to service the facility's clientele during a predetermined shift and only pay trainers additional commissions for sessions completed outside of their scheduled work shift. Individual salaries or commission rates for trainers typically vary based on education, certification, experience, seniority, job performance, and volume of revenue produced. Regardless of the compensation model, it is important that all program costs be considered during planning. General and administrative (G&A) costs for marketing, administrative support, meetings, uniforms, payroll taxes, liability insurance, and continuing education can dramatically effect the profitability of the personal training program. All expenses combined will ultimately decide what the net margins are for the personal training enterprise in a fitness business.

Master classes are a "specialty" offering that serve as a revenue stream and are usually delivered by group exercise instructors. Facilities feature these specialty classes in addition to their standard fare of group exercise classes on their schedule. Typical standard exercise classes may include aerobics, sculpting, step, kickbox-aerobics, mat Pilates, and yoga. Master classes may include "Drums Alive," an exercise class centered around drumming on a balance ball, or sports barre, an exercise class combining sports-oriented agility drills with movements and stretches on a ballet barre. Master classes are marketed individually and separately from the standard group exercise classes, so as not to negatively affect perceived value, making the "extra charge" a fair and expected cost to participate. Group exercise instructors who teach fee-for-service master classes typically receive either a premium rate or a commission above and beyond their regular class pay rate.

THE ROLE OF THE FITNESS "SPECIALIST"

Roles of fitness instructors, group exercise instructors, and personal trainers can be further broken down into specialty areas. These specialties can be one of the many services delivered by the professional or it can be their single focus.

Pilates

Pilates, a specialty initially developed in the early 1900s by Josef Pilates as a rehabilitative and conditioning exercise program for dancers, has become very popular in the last 10 years. It is delivered in both individual and small group sessions, and typically for a premium fee. Traditional Pilates involves the use of specialized equipment (Reformer, Cadillac, etc.), but in the fitness setting, large group classes (*i.e.*, "mat classes") have also become popular, utilizing Pilates-inspired movement techniques. Mat classes are usually part of a facility's standard group exercise class offerings, thus inclusive in most membership-based facilities.

Yoga

Yoga is a common exercise discipline based on Eastern philosophy that is thousands of years old. The most popular mind-body exercise option, yoga involves movement progressions through a series of postures, and has evolved into various styles (*i.e.*, Hatha, Vinyasa, Ashtanga/Power Yoga, Iyengar, Kundalini, Bikram/Hot Yoga) (1). While many yogis deliver private sessions, in most fitness facilities, yoga is delivered in group exercise class sessions as a value-added staple of their mind-body offerings.

Strength and Conditioning Coach

Athletic conditioning has become a popular offering at many fitness facilities in the United States. Performance-based or functional training is the premise in these programs that focus on training progressions designed to enhance athletic performance (Fig. 2-3). Sport-specific performance training parameters include strength, power, balance, speed, agility, and quickness. Because of the widespread participation in youth sports, many of these programs target young participants between the ages of 8 and 18 years. For facilities that have the appropriate space and equipment, such programs are invaluable, since they broaden the facilities' target markets. Sessions are often provided as one-on-one, small-group, and large-group training sessions. Fitness instructors, personal trainers, or group exercise instructors can deliver these sessions, depending on their experience and credentials. In the case of sports performance training, there are NCCA-accredited specialized credentials available (*i.e.*, NSCA-Certified Strength and Conditioning Specialist) that would be most appropriate for the coach. Sports performance training programs are typically fee-for-service offerings. A membership model can also be seen, though seldomly, in unique facilities that can service youth in large numbers.

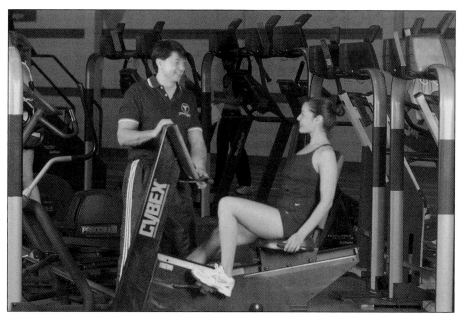

Figure 2-3. A trainer teaching his client proper alignment when using a recumbent bike. Reprinted with permission from ACSM's Resources for the Personal Trainer. 2nd ed. Philadelphia (PA): Lippincott Williams & Wilkins, 2007.

CHAPTER SUMMARY

The three commonly seen fitness professional roles are those of fitness instructor, personal trainer, and group exercise instructor. Each role typically delivers a unique set of services, but there is often a crossover, with each role overlapping and delivering services that would usually be provided by another. Professional experience and credentials typically delineate the roles and the services the individual professional delivers. Basic facility service levels include both value-added services (included with membership costs) and fee-for-service options (fees paid above and beyond membership fees) under a facility's profit center umbrella. The type of service often dictates how the fitness professional is compensated for the delivery of that service.

YOUR RESOURCES

www.ihrsa.org/ — The International Health, Racquet, and Sportsclub Association (IHRSA) is a trade association serving the health and fitness club industry. IHRSA's mission is to grow, protect, and promote the health and fitness industry, and to provide its members with benefits that will help them be more successful. http://clubindustry.com/ — an extensive resource for fitness business professionals.

REFERENCES

1. International Health, Racquet, and Sportsclub Association. *Profiles of Success 2008.* IHRSA, Boston (MA); 2008. p.35.

3 Sales

Chapter Objectives

After reading this chapter, the reader will:

- Understand basic strategies for selling three common fitness services: membership, personal training, and ancillary products and services
- Understand why it is important for the fitness professional acting as salesperson to listen more than talk
- Know how to develop an emotional sale from the initial interview and build value and rapport with the prospect to asking for the sale
- Understand the importance of providing complete and comprehensive sales presentations and diligent follow-up for all prospects that they do not close at their first opportunity

THE FITNESS PROFESSIONAL AS SALESPERSON

There are core competencies that are key to the fitness professional's success. Fitness professionals should be genuine, caring individuals who "like" people and enjoy helping them achieve improvements in health, fitness, or performance. This is something that most career professionals do passionately, without fore-thought. It is why they "get into this business."

There is one core competency, however, that can predict career success and longevity more than almost any other. That is the ability to sell. The fitness professional needs to be proficient with this skill set to "sell" people on exercise and other health-enhancing behaviors. The cost-benefit, in this case, is completely intrinsic, that is, the exerciser must pay in time and effort in order to get his or her planned return on investment: improved health, fitness, or performance. Most fitness professionals are comfortable with selling this targeted behavior. They do it daily, passionately, and without reservation. They often cite pertinent research that supports what they are selling and have no qualms with being persistent to break down the customer's resistance to buying. However, why is it that the minute you introduce a dollar amount that the client must pay in order to receive the benefits, the fitness professional becomes inept?

While there are various theories that might explain this phenomenon, we focus on building value and developing a relationship with the customer to overcome "cost-related" misgivings. Value and relationship selling make it easier for the customer to part with his or her money to pay for the services that he or she is being sold. Value selling requires you to build the specific innate value of the service to the customer, so that you get to the point where it is a bargain and well worth the expense. Relationship selling lowers buying resistance by building rapport and trust. In relationship selling, the salesperson acts as a consultant, helping the customer identify specific needs that may be satisfied by the product or service being sold. A primary goal of relationship selling is to develop a long-term customer relationship that will lead to repeat business. This is crucial in the fitness industry, where referrals and retention are integral to the success of any business. Combining value and relationship selling inevitably builds to an emotional sale. One that focuses not just on what the service will do for the buyer but also how the buyer will feel once achieving his or her projected goal from using the purchased service.

There are three main types of products or services that are most common in the fitness business. The three types are

- Membership sales
- Personal training
- Juice bar/pro shop and other ancillary product and service sales (*e.g.,* massage therapy)

Each of these types has distinctly different approaches to selling. Membership, for one, is usually a cold-market sale. That is, one where the prospect is not already a customer. It is easy for the guest touring your club to walk out without spending a dime and committing to any purchase. Approaching this prospect is vastly different from a personal trainer approaching a member who is already a customer, is spending money every month on dues and other services, and wants to sell the member on his personal training services.

Below, you will find three very distinct approaches to selling each of the common types of products or services. You will note that while each approach is different, there are commonalities that are integrated into each including listening to the prospect, building rapport and trust, matching the prospect's needs to your product or service, identifying the emotional trigger that will ultimately close the prospect, and asking for the sale. Let's look at each approach on a step-by-step basis.

Selling Fitness Club Memberships

Fitness is a service business that has traditionally been sold as a membership in various health club/fitness center environments. Members pay for the privilege of using the facilities, typically on an annual basis, paying for their membership either in monthly installments or on a one-time paid-in-full basis. The fitness professional acting as salesperson should always approach each sales opportunity as a one-time opportunity effectively assuming that if they do not close the prospect at this time, the prospect will not be back. This approach ensures that the salesperson does everything systematically, covering all of the pertinent bases, in order to close the sale. All too often, a salesperson will assume that the prospect will be back to enroll, and as a result not offer a comprehensive presentation to the prospect that would have otherwise resulted in a sale for the salesperson, and a new member for the club.

The Initial Prospect Interview

A unique feature of this type of sale is that prospects are purchasing an intangible, as opposed to buying a "concrete," product — that is, something that they can take, hold, and keep as theirs.

Keeping this in mind, when performing as a salesperson, the fitness professional must go into every sales opportunity understanding that while the prospect is shopping for the privilege of using the facility, their ultimate reason for their interest is rarely the use of the facility, but the desired outcome derived from effectively using the facilities (*i.e.*, weight loss, improved health, etc.). It is crucial for the salesperson to perform an initial prospect interview (see Figure 3-1) to properly set the stage for the sales presentation. The primary objectives of this interview are to develop rapport and trust between the prospect and salesperson, to identify emotional triggers that the salesperson can use to ultimately close the sale, and to qualify the prospect as a true candidate for membership while identifying and resolving objections BEFORE being confronted by them at the close.

[FRONT OF FORM]

Name: _____

Street address: _____

City: _____ ST:_____ Zip: _____

Day phone:_____ Evening phone: _____

Email address: _____

How did you hear about the club?

☐ Member referral: _____

☐ Newspaper advertisement

☐ Flyer or ad in local business

☐ Chamber of Commerce

☐ Physician's referral: Dr._____

☐ Word of mouth

☐ Happen to be in the area

☐ Other: _____

[BACK OF FORM]

- What brings you in today? _____
- How did you hear about the club? _____
- Have you ever been a member of a health club? Where? When? Are you still a member? Why / why not? _____
- What did you like / dislike the most about the club? _____
- What activities did you participate in most? What did you not use? Why? _____
- What ancillary services did you purchase / not purchase? Why / why not? _____
- What did you enjoy the most / least in using these services? _____
- Notes: _____
  _____
  _____

Figure 3-1. The initial prospect interview form is a sample that may be used when performing the initial prospect interview. This intake form provides important information that should help the salesperson identify the prospect's needs, matching those needs to the club's services, and developing the emotional sale of the product or service.

The salesperson wants to get to know the prospect and why the prospect wants to become a member. Some of the most pertinent items of discussion are

- How did the prospect learn about the club? This question can provide powerful information that can help the salesperson close the sale. For example, if the prospect saw a current advertisement with a special offer and a specific call to action, the salesperson can use this information to create urgency when trying to close the sale. If the prospect, instead, simply lives down the street from the facility, the salesperson can emphasize that convenience is one of the main factors that increase a member's success in using their facility and achieving their desired goals. If, instead, the prospect was referred by a member, offering the member's name, the salesperson can refer to the member by name almost making the prospect a "warm-market" membership candidate, further overcoming initial barriers to the sale, building rapport, and dramatically enhancing the chances of closing the sale.
- Has the prospect ever been a member of a health club? Where? When? Are they still a member? Why/why not?
- What did they like/dislike the most about the club?
- What activities did they participate in most? What did they not use? Why?
- What ancillary services did they purchase/not purchase? Why/why not?
- What did they enjoy the most/least in using these services?

These questions provide a history of the prospect's past experiences. If the prospect has never been a health club member, the salesperson knows that they need to gradually educate the prospect so that they have clear expectations of what membership will be like for them. Assess how much "hand-holding" the prospect will need as a member. Point out to the member how the facility's professional staff is there to help them every step of the way, and how personal training can ensure their success. If, instead, the prospect had been a member of several clubs over the years but is presently not an active member anywhere, an assumptive comment like, "So you are looking for a new fitness facility," which prompts a "yes" answer, can take the prospect one step closer toward the close (Figs. 3-2 and 3-3).

This information is also invaluable because it can be used by the salesperson to place the candidate in a member's shoes. That is, if the prospect liked aerobics classes at his or her previous facility, the salesperson might affirm, "Oh yes! We have two group exercise studios, hosting over 100 classes per week, and our members RAVE about our instructors." If the prospect instead was disgusted by a dirty shower at his/her previous facility, the salesperson might say, "Oh, I understand. There is nothing more disgusting than a dirty locker room area. That is why we have full-time attendants whose primary role is to keep our locker rooms immaculately clean. Cleanliness is a priority at our facility."

- What are your fitness goals? Why is achieving these goals important to you? Why now?

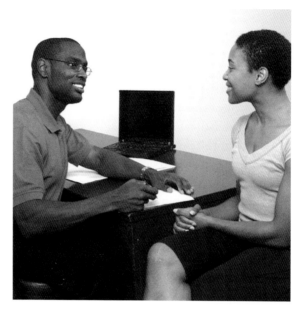

Figure 3-2. Consulting with a client. Be warm, interested and engaged with the client, but most of all LISTEN! Reprinted with permission from ACSM's Resources for the Personal Trainer. 3rd ed. Philadelphia (PA): Lippincott Williams & Wilkins, 2010.

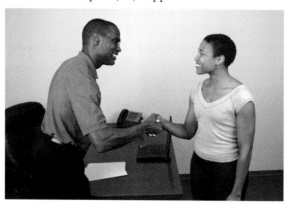

Figure 3-3. Greeting a client. A genuine smile is key! Reprinted with permission from ACSM's Resources for the Personal Trainer. 3rd ed. Philadelphia (PA): Lippincott Williams & Wilkins, 2010.

These "Why" questions can be pivotal in the sales process. Everyone can come up with a "health and/or fitness goal." That is not enough information. The salesperson wants to find out why it is a goal, and to connect achieving the goal with a feeling — that which the prospect will feel upon achieving the goal.

The conversation might sound like this:

Salesperson: "So Bob, you say you want to lose 20 pounds by the end of April. May I ask why?"

Prospect: "Yes, I am going to my 25-year class reunion on May 2nd, and want to look my best."

Salesperson: "That is great. Well, Bob, when you lose those 20 pounds, and become healthier and fitter, and you get all dressed up and walk in the front door at the reunion, and everybody is saying 'Wow! Bob! You look great!' How are you going to feel when that happens?"

Prospect: "I will feel G-R-E-A-T!"

Salesperson: "That's right, Bob. You will feel amazing! And you know what? We do this for our members everyday, and we are going to take you by the hand, develop your customized training program, and get you to the class reunion looking like a movie star!"

The salesperson wants to develop a "list" of positive club attributes that speak directly to the prospect's desires and quell their fears of committing to a membership. In other words, match the prospect with specific facilities, services, and even staff that are aligned with the prospect's specific personal needs and desires. This is a progressive exercise of building value in the prospect's eyes, while lowering the most evident barriers of entry that will result in a membership purchase.

The Presentation

Once the salesperson has learned what specific facility features most interest the prospect, and what objections might present barriers to a commitment and ultimate sale, it is time to build value and personally "connect" the prospect with the facility. The presentation is essentially a personalized guided tour of the facilities where the salesperson has the opportunity to answer the prospect's question, "What's in it for me?" by highlighting the solutions to the member's needs that membership would offer.

What the presentation is not, is a simple tour of all the facilities. Every presentation, while having similarities in flow and features, should have very distinct focuses. If, for example, the prospect has expressed an interest in group exercise classes, it is imperative that you spend some time sharing the class schedule, unique program features, instructors' qualifications, and most importantly how your facility's group exercise program is different than your competitors' offerings. Differentiation is a key element that can make or break a sale.

The presentation should be designed to make the prospect feel as if they were already a member. Provide the prospect with a feeling of belonging. One of the most effective methods of doing this is to introduce the prospect by name to key employees and even members as the salesperson guides the prospect through the facilities. If the prospect has mentioned an interest in personal training, an introduction to the facility's Director of Personal Training is in order. If massage is a service of interest, introduce the prospect to a massage therapist. This is one area where cross-training of staff so they know how to introduce themselves and pique the prospect's interest in their personal services can prove invaluable. The bottom line is that the more faces and names the prospect meets by the end of the presentation, the more "at home" he or she will feel at "closing" time.

Another effective method of making the prospect feel like he or she already "owns" a membership is by having the prospect try a piece of equipment. This minimizes any possible intimidation factor and gives the prospect a feeling of "I can." This empowerment is important, especially with prospects who have a previous history of failed attempts at other facilities. If the prospect expressed interest in building their upper body strength, sit them down on an upright piece of selectorized weight equipment (*i.e.*, chest press), show them how easy it is to set up, and have them try a couple of repetitions. If dealing with daily stress is a major concern for the prospect, point out your yoga or meditation classes, as well as massage therapy. In addition, don't hesitate to educate the prospect throughout the presentation. In this case, explaining how vigorous exercise can help reduce stress and enhance one's ability to deal with daily stressors.

Miniconfirmations

Throughout the presentation there will be several opportunities to "pre-close" the prospect. These are simple leading questions that the prospect will, for the most part, answer with a simple "yes." For example, because of scheduling issues at her former club, a prospect, Mary, has concerns about the facility's babysitting service opening early enough so that she can drop off her toddler, have enough time to make it to her aerobics class, and on the back-end then meet with a personal trainer for a strength training session, before retrieving her toddler and leaving in time to pick up her older child at school. This tight schedule makes it difficult for Mary to imagine being successful and achieving her health and fitness goals. The salesperson could ask the prospect:

Salesperson: "Mary, if I can show you how easy it is for you to take care of your children, and get a great class and strength training session in without wasting time, would that interest you?

Prospect: "Yes."

Salesperson: If you could commit to do this consistently, I can assure you that you will increase your chances of achieving your goals here at our club. Would that make it easy for you to make a commitment and enroll today?

Prospect: "Yes."

The salesperson could then highlight the following:

- "Mary, you are concerned about having enough time to drop off your daughter at our childcare center, the Little Tikes Playroom. You see on our schedule that the Playroom opens at 8:30 am every morning. This gives you

30 minutes to sign your daughter into the Playroom, get her settled, and get yourself to the group exercise class of your choice. Do you think you can do that?" *prompted response: "Yes."*

- "If you look at our class schedule, Mary, most weekend mornings we offer three different classes starting promptly at 9 am. We offer three classes at the same time to keep any one class from overcrowding, so you are assured a spot in any of these classes. Given the variety of classes offered at the time, don't you think you can choose a class at that time that you will enjoy?" *prompted response: "Yes."*
- "I know, Mary, that you are afraid that we won't be able to accommodate you with a training appointment after class. If you look here at our Personal Trainers' Bios Board, which lists all of our certified trainers along with their education, credentials, and training specialties, you can see we have a great roster of professional, qualified, and experienced trainers, and several are available to take care of you between 10 and 11 am. Don't you think that we will be able to match you up with a trainer of your choice at your convenience after class?" *prompted response: "Yes."*
- "So, on any given weekday we can assure you enough time to drop off your daughter, get to a great class, followed by a personal training session, and then have enough time to get your daughter at our childcare center before it closes at noon, and leave to pick up your son at school. Based on your personal goals, and tight schedule, doesn't that sound like the perfect solution for you? *prompted response: "Yes."*

The beauty of this type of progressive approach is that the salesperson is eliminating objections ahead of time, prior to the close. This is why the information gathered at the initial interview is crucial, since it sets up the rest of the presentation, and will provide the salesperson the ammunition needed to target emotional triggers and fend off objections.

The Close

After the presentation, the salesperson should return to where the initial interview was conducted, or to a designated location in the club that provides some privacy without intimidating the prospect. The purpose of the close is to highlight the specific points of value that membership offers the prospect, to present the membership options highlighting the best options for the prospect, and to ask for the sale. During the close, the salesperson will review with the prospect their fitness goals and any other positive attributes of being a club member (*i.e.*, convenience, hours, desired facilities and services, etc.). The salesperson will then review each of the miniconfirmations that came up during the presentation and answer any remaining questions, followed by a presentation of rates and payment options.

It is important to present any membership options as "either/or" options (*i.e.*, the paid-in-full or monthly installment option), as opposed to a "yes or no" option.

Hesitation on the prospect's part will usually be presented as objections, which is why it's important to try to get these out in the open early during the initial interview and presentation so as to disarm the prospect, and minimize objections at the time of the close. The most popular objections are

- Time — "I don't have enough time to exercise." Asking the right questions (as in the case above with Mary, who had a tight schedule), or even as simple as, "When do you see yourself coming into the club to exercise?" Or saying, "We are open from 5 am every morning until 11 pm every night. Don't you think you can commit to 30–60 minutes 3 days per week to achieve your goals, and looking great at your class reunion? (In this case, the salesperson is targeting the prospect's emotional trigger).
- Significant other — "I have to check with my husband." Finding out early in the interview if the prospect has a support system (*i.e.*, spouse, significant other) who will support his or her desire to achieve his or her health and fitness goals is a good approach to squashing this common objection.
- Money — "It is more than I expected to spend." Money objections can often be fended off by identifying whether it is the price or the payment schedule that is the problem. An annual membership for $800 might sound overwhelming to a prospect, but broken into 12 installments of $69 per month, it suddenly becomes feasible, even if they are paying a little bit more ($828). Some prospects feel that they don't want to pay the little bit extra by taking the installment plan. Other prospects do not like using the electronic fund transfer payment programs used by most clubs, and want to maintain control over their payments. Using a credit card gives the prospect the option to pay the $800 on his or her schedule and, since it is a close-ended contract, gives the salesperson the option of manipulating the membership term to enhance the call to action. That is, "OK, Bob, enroll now, paying-in-full with your credit card, and I will add an additional month to your membership free of charge. That is a cost of about $61 per month, cheaper than our monthly installment plan, and you are in complete control of how and when you pay."
- Money-back guarantee — This is a tactic that has come into vogue over the last 10 years. These days, many consumers know that even if they sign on the dotted line today, they will likely have a couple of days to change their mind, receive a full refund of any payments initially made, and be free of any time commitment made at the time of signing. This is typically known as the "Buyer's Remorse" law and in most states allows for cancellation of a contract within 3 days of signing. Some businesses actually extend this no-penalty period to a 15- or even 30-day period. The benefit is obviously

lowering the risk of entry for the members. The risk to the club is that if they don't deliver on the new member's expectations within the first few weeks of their membership, the member is free to walk away. Once again, it is important that the staff understand that they need to "shine" everyday with every member, because if they drop the ball, it can mean losing a member. It is important to front-load your fitness programming, as well, since it will help engage the new member, keeping them active and busy in various areas of the club during the first few weeks of their membership.

The "Be-back"

Every membership prospect who says "no" becomes a "future prospect." The salesperson should maintain a database or "tickler file" of contact and personal information (*i.e.*, likes, dislikes, occupation, etc.) of these prospects for future contacts, always looking for the opportunity to pitch membership and ask for a sale. The salesperson should continue to "drip" or regularly communicate via every available vehicle (in person, on phone, by e-mail or snail-mail, etc.) with the prospect. Scanning clips of fitness articles that the prospect might be interested in and e-mailing them to the prospect, e-mailing a web-based link to a pertinent Web site, or even a press release with the fitness facility's current programs are all examples of how to effectively "drip" on prospects to build membership value. The most important thing is to keep regular tabs with the prospect so that when the time comes for the prospect to seriously consider enrollment, your facility naturally comes to mind.

Selling Personal Training

Personal trainers, in general, are not known for their "selling skills," but the most successful trainers are. Too often, personal trainers focus their "sales" efforts on creating signs, flyers, and brochures, hoping that clients will flock to them for training. The mistake they make is that such efforts are "low-percentage" marketing activities that offer a low return on their investment of time, money, and effort. In addition, these activities do not close the sale for the personal trainer. They only weed out potential prospects for the personal trainer's services, and the trainer is depending on the client to respond to the marketing piece. The key to sales success is for the personal trainer to use the resources available to him or her, proactively cultivate his or her warm-market leads or "suspects" to convert them into prospects, and finally ask the prospect for the sale.

Before going into the sales process, let us first define what a "sale" is. A sale is simply an agreement — a quid pro quo — between the personal trainer, the client, and, at times, the facility where the training sessions will take place. A sale is not an imposition on the client. All too often, a trainer is "apologetic" when asking for the sale. In actuality, every sale is a win-win situation, because everyone involved positions themselves to get what they want. The client is securing the direction, expertise, or motivation they desire, and the personal trainer is contracting his professional services. The ingredient needed to fulfill the sale is commitment. The client must commit to what they agreed to at the point of sale (*i.e.*, showing up prepared for the training session at the scheduled time), and the personal trainer must commit to deliver on his service "promise" to the client (*i.e.*, delivering a safe, individualized, goal-oriented workout).

In the gym or fitness center environment, the personal trainer's primary source of business is the membership base. This captive audience is the personal trainer's main resource for "suspects." It is important for the personal trainer to establish himself or herself as an expert and to build rapport with the members. This creates a warm market for the trainer to target, market to, and ultimately to ask for the sale.

Before approaching members on the exercise floor, the personal trainer should have a clear understanding of what his or her objective is and what value he or she brings to the table. It is important to be empathetic and see things through the eyes of the member. Why should the member consider personal training? What is in it for the member? The personal trainer should know what the benefits of personal training are to the client (see Box 3.1).

BOX 3.1	**BENEFITS OF PERSONAL TRAINING**

- Client achieves results more quickly
- Reduces the risk of injury to the client
- Increases the client's motivational levels
- Provides more focused workouts for the client
- Utilizes client's time more efficiently

The trainer needs to be aware of the prospect's questions and concerns. What are the prospect's perceptions? Will personal training help get the participant more fit? Will it help them look better? Will it help them be healthier? These are all valuable benefits and perceived outcomes for the participant, but, ultimately, even if the prospect perceives these outcomes as real, they still might not make the commitment to purchase training sessions. Why? It is because it is all about the prospect's emotions. The trainer must consider how the prospect feels about their goals, and how they will feel when they fulfill them.

Effective sales generation is simply a step-by-step process. Below is a simple approach, perfect for a facility-based personal trainer. It will ensure success, regardless of the personal trainer's salesmanship (1).

Making Contact — *"Getting his foot in the door"*

A personal trainer needs to proactively approach a facility member or client as they are exercising on the gym floor. They should greet the member with a smile and offer their expertise based on their observations of the member.
Sample "openings":

- "Hi! May I help you with your exercise program?"
- "Hey Mark, let me show you a more effective way to do this exercise."
- "Hello Linda, I noticed you're really focusing on your lower body. Can I show you a great new combination of exercises for your hips and thighs?"

Building Rapport — "Trust me?" *Yes!!!*

A personal trainer must build rapport and trust so that the prospect believes in him and his ability to help the client achieve his goals. A personal trainer builds trust by taking a personal interest in the prospect, making mental notes of the prospects likes, dislikes, or personal information that the prospect may have shared with the trainer.
Sample "blurbs":

- "Hi John, you haven't been here since before Thanksgiving..."
- "Hello Marie, how was your business trip?"
- "Hi Jessica, did your daughter decide between colleges?"

Assessing Need — *"shut up and listen!!!"*

The best salespersons are seldom the best talkers — they're usually the best listeners. He must key into *"What's in it for the prospect?"* He must not just focus on "what" the prospect wants, but also learn *why* the prospect wants it.

The Tease

This is how the personal trainer continues to build trust and demonstrate and build his value. The most effective way to do this is by "training the prospect" through a set or two of exercise. It will be clear to the prospect what the difference is between working with the trainer and working on their own.

Presenting a Winning Proposition — *Asking for the Sale*

The personal trainer must present a winning solution to the prospect's need, before asking for the sale. This "frames" the pitch so that the prospect responds affirmatively when asked for the sale.

- "You really want to lose the 10 pounds by your High School Reunion in June, don't you?"
- "If I can show you how I can help you reach your goal, would that interest you?"

The Close

The personal trainer should give the prospect "either/or" choices, never "yes" or "no."

Sample "yes or no" proposal: "Marie, would you like to set up a training appointment?"

Sample "either/or" proposal: "Marie, you're usually here in the morning, I'm available to help you any two mornings per week at 6 am or 7 am. Which works best for you?"

Giving the prospect a choice between two "yeses" increases the likelihood that the trainer will close the sale.

The Fallback — *"The Tickler File"*

Every prospect who says "no" becomes a "future prospect." The personal trainer should maintain a database of contact and personal information (*i.e.*, likes, dislikes, occupation, etc.) of these prospects for further rapport building, always looking for the opportunity to once again ask for the sale. The trainer should continue to deliver service (*i.e.*, assistance on the training floor) or communicate via every available vehicle (in person, on phone, by e-mail, etc.), increasing his value as a trainer. Photocopying clips of fitness articles that the prospect might be interested in and providing them for the client, e-mailing a web-based link to a pertinent Web site, or even a press release with the trainer's own "success story" are all examples of how to effectively "drip" on prospects to build a trainer's value. The personal trainer in a fitness center setting should also do whatever he can to keep the prospect coming in to work out, even if the prospect continues to train on his own. Doing so helps to maintain the trainer's "warm market," so that the prospect remains a prospect, and is also a source of referrals to the trainer.

Keep in mind: *It's a "numbers game"*

An insurance company study conducted several years back showed that even the worst approach to selling can be successful if the salesperson simply goes through the numbers and "keeps asking" (see Box 3.2).

Selling Personal Training in a Studio Setting

Selling training services in a studio setting is similar to selling memberships in the health club setting. The prospect is not a current customer, and is likely a cold-market opportunity. The initial interview is designed, again, to build rapport, gather information, and establish the prospect's needs and how training at your studio satisfies those needs.

In the studio setting, the initial interview is typically followed by either a physical assessment or sample workout. Because of this "active" component, some preactivity screening is commonly included in the initial interview. Using

| BOX 3.2 | **THE FITNESS FACILITY–BASED TRAINER'S SALES CHECKLIST** |

- Be proactive. Approach prospects and always remember to smile — act as if — be positive and upbeat, no matter how bad a day you are having
- Top priority is to build rapport — to develop a relationship of mutual trust and confidence
- Sell benefits of personal training but key into how they'll feel when achieving those benefits
- Be empathetic — see their world as if it were your own
- Be genuine — exude sincerity
- Be warm — treat prospects with respect
- It's a win-win situation!
    - Clients — take control of their goals by hiring an expert's assistance
    - Trainers — practice their profession, increase their earning potential, and add valuable experience, which enhances their value to the employer or facility and the fitness industry in general
    - The facility enhances the service delivered to the client by providing 1-on-1 management of members
- You must ask for the sale! — It is a numbers game. The more prospects you ask, the more sales you'll make. "You never make the shots you don't take" (Wayne Gretzky)

a simple tool like a Par-Q can indicate whether medical clearance is needed or recommended. There is nothing more powerful in getting a commitment than having a prospect who answers "yes" on the Par-Q and receives medical clearance with a specific recommendation from his or her physician to exercise.
Typical assessments may include

- Total body weight — Everyone's common "measuring stick" and most common goal or reason to start an exercise program.
- Body composition/body fat% — Demystifying body composition for the prospect can put you in the "expert's seat." While skinfold measurements are simple to do, a handheld bioimpedence analyzer is simple, fast, and noninvasive. This is important, especially when measuring a prospect of the opposite gender, since it will be less intimidating for the more modest prospects. It can also provide a perception of "high-tech," which piggybacks closely to "state-of-the-art," which makes another positive statement about you and your studio.
- Body mass index and/or waist-hip ratio — Addresses obesity as a health risk, and body fat distribution. Most consumers have heard that it's better

to be a pear than an apple. This along with most of these body fatness-related measurements speak emotionally to most Americans these days, as most of us are overweight, want to lose weight, and at least recognize the connection between physical exercise and weight loss.

- Waist circumference measurement — Indicates health risk, and is a powerful reality check, especially for male prospects.
- Resting heart rate — A high resting heart rate is understood by most people as "not good." Regular exercise can help lower it to a more efficient resting rate — an obvious benefit of training with you.
- Resting blood pressure — Many people are hypertensive and don't even know it.
- Basic postural analysis — This is a simple assessment of standing posture. Observing forward head with rounded shoulders, for example, can indicate tight chest muscles, which is common in anyone whose day is spent in front of a computer in an office setting. A protruding abdominal wall ("big belly") indicates an abnormal forward pelvic tilt and tight lower back muscles, which can exacerbate low back pain. Reporting these findings to the prospect might lead them to connect a stiff neck or low back ache to the postural deviations. If you can present a training program that can help alleviate these conditions, consider it a miniclose.

Once the assessment or sample workout is completed, the prospect and salesperson should return to the location where they met for the initial interview, or sit in a designated quiet, private area, where they can speak candidly about what observations were made, how personal training at the studio can "fix" these findings, and how great the client will feel after "fixing" them. Then, they can discuss training plan costs. Many studios offer special pricing for new clients' initial packages. This practice often lowers the barrier of entry for new clients who have not committed to the studio or experienced any benefits of training as yet.

Conversion Time

The chapter on Marketing will delve deeper into the member/client acquisition process, but it is essential to understand that the process by which a suspect

BOX 3.3	Keep in mind that discounting can be a very tricky thing. Lowering your rates can devalue your services. You are usually better off not discounting price and providing value-added benefits for large purchases (*i.e.*, gift with purchase: gym apparel with large package of personal training sessions, or a bundle of free services for immediate call-to-action responses like do-it-now special).

becomes a member or client can sometimes take quite some time. As leads find their way into your sales pipeline, and become a prospect, it can take weeks or months to convert the prospect into a client. The studio trainer should drip and regularly follow-up with every training prospect who goes through your sales presentation process. If several weeks have passed since the original presentation, including an assessment, insist on repeating the complete assessment or sample workout, since their body can change over time, and you need to benchmark their actual starting point. Then you can simply follow your well-rehearsed proven sales system, provide the prospect optimal value, and, once again, ask for the sale.

Selling Ancillary Services and Products

Ancillary services like massage therapy, juice bar drinks and smoothies, along with Pro Shop equipment and apparel fall into this sales category. Cross-selling and program packaging are two ways to drive ancillary sales.

Many facilities offer a handful of gifts-with-purchase for new membership enrollees. This is an example of cross-selling. A new member will typically pay an initiation or enrollment fee upon enrollment. This fee will offset the costs of acquisition (finding the member and cost of converting him from suspect, to prospect, to member) as well as any costs associated with the gift-with-purchase. When the new member enrolls, he or she might receive a handful of gift certificates or coupons entitling him or her to a protein shake at the juice bar, a 30-minute chair massage, a basic food plan from the club nutritionist, and the like. These "gifts" introduce the new member to a sampling of some of the club's ancillary services, and give the service provider an opportunity to convert the member into a regular customer.

Program packaging integrates services, providing for a natural "upsell" that can be a logical part of any package. For example, exercise science has shown that super-compensation is the process by which a body exercises and, through recovery and adaptation, becomes "more fit" as a result. The super-compensation or

---

BOX 3.4

It is important, regardless of what you are selling, to make sure that you completely cross-train your staff so that all employees understand the basics of any programs running concurrently in your club, and can effectively promote, sell, or in the very least answer simple questions about the programs and know who to refer prospects to. If you can devise a system that accurately measures how many referrals, leads, or sales of a specific program or item come directly from a unique frontline employee, a reward and staff recognition system can be very motivating, providing a positive incentive for the employee to "talk up" your products and services.

improvement phase does not happen during a workout, but instead between workouts. It has also been established that anything that enhances recovery from a workout will enhance the resulting super-compensation. So it becomes a natural approach to combine exercise or an optimal training stimulus (personal training) with nutrition or "refueling the system" (juice bar/supplements) and recuperation or "repairing the system" (massage therapy). One program feeds the other and supporting marketing or conditioning packages can include all three or call for the purchase of the additional complementary service upon using either of the other two services. Combining these programs in this way makes sense to the consumer, and thus, closing the member is less difficult.

CHAPTER SUMMARY

This chapter reviews the three most common sales items in the fitness industry: membership, personal training, and ancillary products and services. It presents three distinct strategies to sell these services, noting the importance of listening to the prospect's unique needs and goals to maximize the closing opportunity and notes the importance of cross-training your employees, so they are thoroughly aware of and can help promote your products and services.

YOUR RESOURCES

Act! is an example of a Contact and Customer Relationship Management Software program that is reasonably priced, easy to use, and provides a robust array of tools to help track and communicate with your prospects. It makes for an ideal "tickler file." This business application is available at http://www.act.com/

REFERENCES

1. American College of Sports Medicine. *ACSM's Resources for the Personal Trainer*. 2nd ed. Baltimore (MD): Lippincott, Williams, & Wilkins, 2007. p. 482.

Marketing

Chapter Objectives

After reading this chapter, the reader will:

- Understand the basics of external and internal marketing as it relates to a health and fitness business
- Understand several marketing tactics, from basic advertising to guerilla marketing tactics
- Understand the basics of e-marketing strategies
- Be able to collect basic marketing outcomes data and integrate it with their sales activities

MARKETING FITNESS

Merriam-Webster's defines marketing as the act, process, or technique of promoting, selling, and distributing a product or service (1). The term marketing has been used in place of other actions in the process of taking a product or service from production to its actual sale. For the purposes of this chapter, we will focus on marketing as any process whose primary objective is to find and identify potential buyers (aka "leads") of your health- and fitness-related products and services. These potential clients may be converted to "prospects" (aka "qualified" leads), and even a step further into paying customers.

Marketing is how you "get the word out." Whether you are announcing the introduction of a new product or service, establishing or developing your brand, or spreading the news of a seasonal offering, the ultimate goal of all marketing is to bring customers, in most cases, members, or clients in the door.

Types of Marketing

Internal Marketing

In the health and fitness business, especially when selling ancillary services like personal training or spa services to those who are already customers, you are targeting a "captive" audience. Your marketing in this case is aimed at your current facility members or clients, who are "inside your walls." Marketing that targets this group is known as internal marketing. The approach and marketing techniques will often be different when recruiting current customers to purchase more services than when the goal is to attract new members/clients.

Common media for internal marketing include
Signs and flyers

- Post signs and provide access to flyers (aka "takeaways") in highly trafficked areas. These can be of the traditional "paper" kind, or if there is an appropriate wall or screen in a strategic location, consider setting up a laptop and projector with a PowerPoint slideshow loop that includes current promotions.
- Bulletin boards are useful, since they provide a specific place for signs, which can keep things "neat" and orderly, and when used effectively can actually draw members who want to get program information, who will also see the internal promotional signs.
- Walking billboards — staff can dress in promotional attire to increase member awareness. They can wear printed t-shirts or even "Ask me about..." buttons to get a customer's attention and prompt a conversation about the current promotion. For example, what can a fitness facility do to promote a special personal training with a "beach body" or "get in shape for summer" theme? If the facility typically has its staff in navy blue polo shirts — or any other basic uniform, for that matter — walking in and seeing the entire staff wearing Hawaiian shirts is an instant attention grabber. Couple that with cross-promotions including a "sunless tan" spa treatment and complimentary tropical smoothie shots at the juice bar, and members will buzz.

Audiovisual/e-media

- Simple public address announcements
- Periodic announcements as part of club audio/ambient music system
- Closed-circuit/private broadcast television systems (*e.g.*, ClubCom; see Box 4.1)

Staff contests

- This is a creative way to cross-train staff while providing them an incentive to take advantage of each employee's "warm market," or the people they each have personal rapport with. Before starting any promotional event, provide staff with all of the pertinent information and an incentive or prize. At the end of the promotion, whether it's a week, a month, or a quarter, the employee with the most sales, referrals, points, etc. wins the prize. The prize can be as simple as a juice bar gift card to movie tickets to a local theatre, or depending on the amount of sales and profit margin, a monetary bonus may be appropriate.

External Marketing

Marketing that targets a demographic that is "outside your walls" (*i.e.*, nonmembers) is known as external marketing. Because this target audience is not presently

---

BOX 4.1 **CLUBCOM**

ClubCom constructs and operates private television networks for targeted health club and other audiences. Health Club management can provide ClubCom with specific information about their membership demographics, along with special internal promotions (*i.e.*, member referrals, personal training packages, juice bar promos), and they will broadcast targeted programming throughout the club.

ClubCom has a wide variety of music video and other content that they broadcast to entertain your club members. Interspersed between videos, you can communicate with your audience instantly through on-screen video text messaging, internal promotions, and brand message reinforcement.

ClubCom also makes it easy for the club owner-operator to participate in local, regional, and national advertising revenue-earning opportunities. A local chiropractor or a chain of health food stores or even supermarkets might choose to advertise to your members. Naturally, the club would earn a portion of the fee paid by the advertiser.

a member/client, they are considered a "cold market," and the approach is likely to be different. The goal is to attract leads from the facility's demographic and geographical area to simply inquire by phone, e-media, or in person about memberships and/or other member/client services.

Common media for external marketing include

Advertising

- Print ads
- Television/cable TV/radio
- Direct mail
- E-mail marketing/Web site/smart phones/texts/tweets/Facebook/other

Guerilla marketing or "nontraditional" advertising vehicles

- Business cards/flyers or brochure distribution
- Ad displays at strategic venues (see Figures 4-1 to 4-3)
- Prescription pads for local physicians (see Your Resources — "Exercise is Medicine")
- Cross-marketing with local businesses
- Gift certificate donations to local schools/boosters fund-raisers

Marketing Personal Training and Fitness Services

The personal training market includes different groups of people with varying needs. A market niche represents a client group with similar needs and goals. Trainers often choose to focus their marketing efforts on one or several of these groups. For example, a trainer may select their niche market based on the following:

- Client type, for example, gender, age, fitness level, health needs, etc.
- Training needs, for example, sport-specific training, prenatal fitness, group training, etc.
- Training location, for example, in-home training, health club training, sport location training, etc.
- Trainers should ask the following questions when selecting their market niches:
  1. What is the potential for income with this market?
  2. Is this market readily accessible in my geographic area?
  3. Does this market fit well with my training skills and interest?
  4. Can I highlight my knowledge, services, certifications, skills, etc. in such a way to reach this market as my clientele?

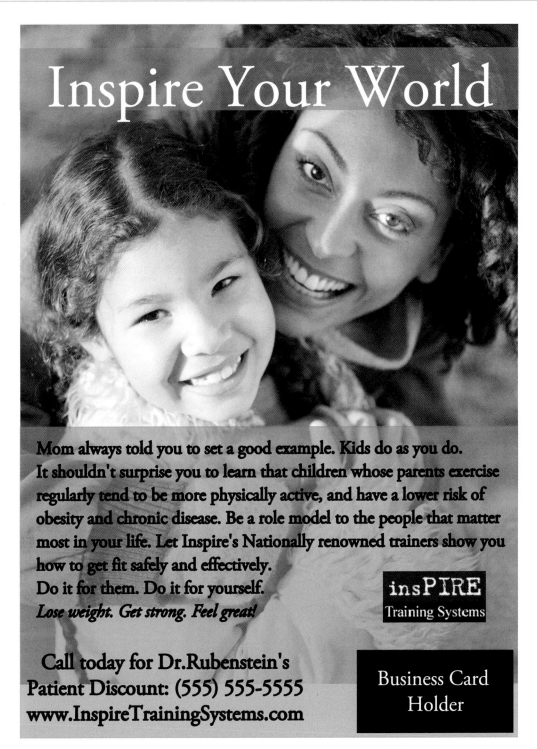

Figure 4-1. Inspire your world display ad with business card or trifold flyer takeaway. This is a sample display ad for use in a gynecologist's office waiting room. It targets women with children, urging them to be a positive role model for their children.

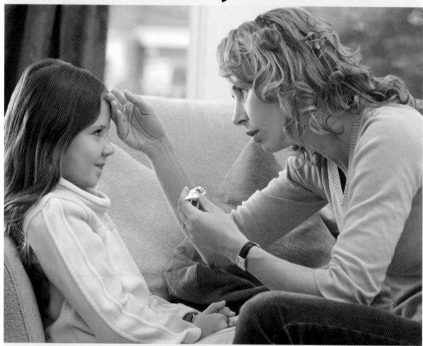

You care for your world.

Don't forget you are in it.

Isn't it time you do something for yourself? Inspire will take care of you. Our Nationally renowned trainers will help you get in the best shape of your life. Let Inspire show you how. Besides, if you don't take care of yourself, you won't be taking care of anyone else. *Lose weight. Get strong. Feel great!*

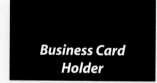

insPIRE
Training Systems

Call today for Dr. Fried's Patient Discount: (555) 555-5555 www.InspireTrainingSystems.com

Business Card Holder

Figure 4-2. Caregiver display ad with business card or trifold flyer takeaway. This is a sample display ad for use in a pediatrician's office waiting room. It target's mothers who care for their kids, putting their own needs aside, urging them to exercise so they can stay healthy enough to continue to care for their family. Note that both ads in Figures 4.1 and 4.2 provide a personalized call to action offering a special discount for their physician's patients. This serves a couple of purposes. It is a simple call to action, and implies an endorsement from the physician, which you have indeed received prior to placing the display ad in the waiting room. It also might lead to an inquiry by the patient to the physician, which is one of the "strongest" referral sources you will ever have. You have of course met with the physician in advance and provided a prescription pad for your services, which makes it easy for him or her to refer the patient.

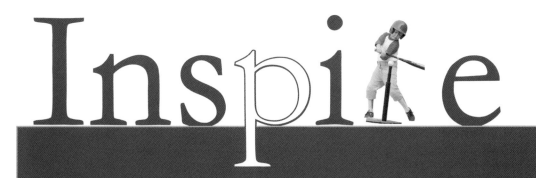

inspire *v. - to stimulate (a person) and create activity*

Whether you are All-State, All-County, or simply trying to make the team, we will **inspire** you to achieve your best. Our tailored approach to performance enhancement will help you take your game to a whole new level.

Hit for Power.
Take the extra base.
Score more runs.
Be your best!

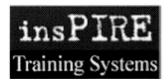

Call today!
Pre-Season Special ends soon!
(555) 555-5555 or go to:
www.InspireTrainingSystems.com

Business
Card
Holder

Figure 4-3. Baseball conditioning display ad with business card or trifold flyer takeaway. It is designed for display at a baseball instruction school, or recreation center that might host a baseball league or several teams. The ad highlights the business's brand, implies a unique sales proposition (*i.e.*, "tailored approach"), then emphasizes the benefits to the client, and provides a time-sensitive call to action.

One of the best ways for personal trainers to market their services is to ask for referrals from satisfied clients. Trainers sometimes are hesitant to do this, but if they truly believe that a client has received great benefits from working with them, then they will want other potential clients to also receive the benefit of working with them. Other ways of marketing personal training include volunteering to speak at community events and organizations and networking with other business professionals in the community. Advertising in the phone book, the newspaper, and by direct mail can be costly and may not provide a good return on the investment. Establishing a Web site and profiling a trainer's style and qualifications is another good approach for marketing and staying competitive in the personal training business (2).

Personal training businesses use a variety of strategies to attract clients. Among the more popular strategies are the following:

1. Client referral

- The focus is on generating prospects and clients.
- The process involves existing clients providing the names of potential new clients.
- Clients are provided with referral cards to hand in the names of prospects.
- Incentives are typically given to present members/clients for providing referrals.
- It is usually an ongoing strategy.
- This approach is the most focused strategy.

2. Lead boxes

- This strategy primarily serves as a source for leads (names).
- The boxes are placed in business locations that tend to serve customer bases that are demographically similar to the targeted audiences.
- Businesses are given awards for allowing the lead boxes to be placed in their locales.
- This strategy might not yield you a high direct return but will provide you with a network of local business owners and managers to cross-market with.

3. Advertising

- In general, this strategy is designed to build brand recognition in the marketplace, enhance the image of the organization, create leads, or occasionally generate prospects.

- This technique is a shotgun approach to reaching clients compared to more targeted methods such as direct mail.
- Cable television, radio, newspapers, billboards, and external or internal signage are examples of this method.
- The most effective type of advertising for generating leads or prospects provides a "call to action," and typically creates urgency by establishing a deadline, for example, "Enroll today and receive a $50 gift card. Offer expires May 30, 2011."
- It is important to know your marketing target niche before the advertising medium is selected.
- This, like most shotgun approaches, is likely to yield a low percent return, but costs will dictate actual return on investment (ROI).

4. Alliances with homeowner associations (HOAs) and realtors

- This strategy is a good source for qualified leads and prospects. HOAs and realtors whose customers match the organization's target market should be engaged in the process.
- HOAs and realtors can provide the names of new people in the area.
- The strategy involves providing the HOAs or realtors a certificate or letter to give to customers that offers some complimentary service (*i.e.*, training session or preactivity screening and goals analysis).

5. Direct mail

- This strategy is primarily a technique for creating leads or turning leads into prospects.
- This method is a more focused technique than advertising.
- Direct mail lists from agencies should be used. Very targeted lists (*i.e.*, zip codes or even specific delivery routes) can be obtained to best match the desired market area and demographics of the target audience (see Box 4.2).
- The piece that is mailed is typically simple, with an attention-grabbing call to action, and normally incorporates an incentive to create urgency and generate an action response.
- This method tends to be costly, with a typical low rate of return.

6. Community involvement

- This strategy focuses on creating relationships to uncover prospects.
- The technique involves creating a specific image in the community and becoming a recognized professional in the community.

BOX 4.2	**THE FREE SEMINAR STRATEGY**

The Free Seminar has been a mainstay of many direct sales and marketing companies for years. It is simple, can be a low-cost marketing strategy, and will give you access to prospects in your demographic area to either sell or follow-up the market and sell in the future. It involves hosting or simply delivering a presentation as part of a related event. It is a great way to develop your name and business brand in the community. It is an opportunity for you to share your expertise with your target market, establishing yourself as a local expert, promote a current program or general business services, and collect contact information from all of the attendees. Here is a step-by-step checklist to follow when hosting a Free Seminar:

- Identify an informational need that you can fulfill in a brief presentation, and that your services resolve for your customers. "How-to" themes are ideal. If you are unsure what to choose as your theme, ask your current customers what information is important to their success that people like them want to know. If you are a trainer who works with young soccer players, whose coaches are always trying to improve their players' agility, try this: How to Improve Your Soccer Team's Speed and Quickness to Score More Goals and Win More Games.

- Identify your target niches. In this case, I would choose to target parents and coaches of youth soccer players. First, work your "inner circle" and then expand it to reach a larger similar group of contacts. First, list out who you already know within this group, and then ask them who else you should reach out to and invite to this special event. Add all such leads to your permanent leads database.

- Secure a location, date, and time for your presentation.

- List out any equipment or "hardware" that you might need for your presentation, for example, chairs and tables, if needed. If you plan on developing a PowerPoint file for your presentation, decide if you need a laptop, projector, and screen to deliver it. Will you be providing presentation handouts (recommended) for your attendees? Will you provide a "free gift" like a sample training program to all who attend? Such takeaways can be "promised" at the event in exchange for attendees e-mail addresses and completed session evaluation forms. See "e-marketing" below for more detailed e-mail–based marketing tactics.

- Promote your event both internally and externally. Send out your invitations either by snail mail or e-mail. Post the event on your business homepage, and any Web 2.0 networking pages (*i.e.*, Facebook, My Space, Twitter), and link them to a promotional page that describes the event and includes a call to action offering your free gift to all registrants who attend. Provide a "Reservation Form" page where visitors can reserve a seat at the event. This ensures that you collect prospects' contact information whether or not they actually attend your seminar. Develop and distribute a Press Release via a public relations distribution service and/or directly to your local media contacts.

- Prepare an information packet for all attendees that includes information on your programs, pricing, and any current promo that you want to highlight for this target market. Also have a registration form for attendees' contact information and enrollment forms for anyone who wants to sign up for a "Trial Session" or another complimentary service offer you might want to serve up as a "carrot."
- Host/present your seminar. Following your presentation, network with attendees every chance you get. Collect contact information on anyone who has not, as yet, provided their information. Present, pitch, and enroll prospects for a trial session.
- Ensure that all registrants and attendees have been entered into your database, and follow-up accordingly.
- Repeat the process outlined above monthly to different market niches, and or quarterly to the same niches. Map out a 12-month plan of seminars for future promotions.

- An example of this approach is to become active in community organizations, such as the local chambers of commerce, the Rotary, church groups, and so on.
- Another option is to host community events in the training facility or sponsor community events at other locations.
- This strategy is ideal for service- and relationship-driven businesses like personal training.

7. Reputation management

- This strategy is used to enhance the public image of the organization.
- Over time, this approach can be a great source for prospects.
- The technique involves developing a press kit on the trainer or the business as a whole (*e.g.*, a background, fact sheet).
- This strategy requires establishing positive relationships with the local media.
- The approach requires regularly issuing press releases of human interest involving the club and following up with the media.

8. Promotional materials

- This strategy is normally used to assist converting leads to prospects or prospects to members.

- The materials are designed to create a positive image of the business and to help educate consumers on your services in general, your business, and its trainers, and other services.
- Web sites, print brochures, and video brochures are examples of this technique.
- These materials are normally given to leads and more often to prospects.

9. Strategic alliances

- This strategy is designed to create partnerships between businesses and organizations with similar target audiences.
- This technique is good at bringing in leads and prospects.
- The approach involves cross-marketing between the businesses. For example, a personal trainer might partner with a home fitness equipment retailer. Offering equipment purchasers a complimentary "orientation to the purchased equipment," with the objective to convert them into personal training clients. The retailer has a "value-added service" (the trainer), which might be an inducement for the customer to purchase the equipment.
- The customers of each business become potential customers for the other partner (alliance group) (1).

E-Marketing

Recent advances in e-marketing technology and its mainstream use require that we take a close look at how to use this technique. The Internet has revolutionized how we communicate and has given rise to many new vehicles that can serve as optimal marketing tools.

Business Web Site

These days, it is rare to find any business that does not have a presence on the Internet — at the very least an informational homepage with contact info. There are many rules that web designers might follow when developing a business Web site. For our purposes, however, understand that the primary marketing goal of a business Web site is acquiring leads, gathering contact information, and funneling these leads into the sales pipeline. It is the sales team's job (or yours, if you are a "one-man-show") to convert leads into prospects, and then members/clients.

There are many options to designing and developing a business Web site. Whether the business uses a professional designer or one of the many online or PC-based design options available, make sure that it includes

- A clear description of the business and core services — Describe the business and why the customer should choose it over another option.

- Contact information — Business address(es), telephone numbers, and e-mail address(es).
- Call to action — Why the lead should call: *"Call today to take advantage of our New Year's Special!"* or *"Contact us today to let us know you saw us on the web, and ask for your special prize!"* — This tactic prompts the collection of their contact information and automatically gives you the marketing source of the lead: the Web site. Many Web sites will bring all potential customers to a specific landing page, sometimes known as a "squeeze" page that offers the customer something of interest in return for their e-mail address or other contact information.

Search Engine Optimization

One of the first things that every new company did only 10 years ago was to establish their business listing in the yellow pages and other such business directories. Small display ads would increase the probability that potential customers would find your business when they looked in the directory for your goods and services. With the advent, popularity, and ease of use of web-based search engines (Google, Yahoo, AOL Search, etc.), the "big books" or yellow pages have become obsolete, and in many markets are no longer published. Search engines place your business and those of your competitors at your customers' fingertips. There are just a few simple things you must do to make sure that when a customer searches for your goods and services, they find you before your competition.

The "big" search engines like Google, Yahoo, and Bing encourage business owners to register and to log on to their business solution areas and to then provide specific information about their business. This can include everything from unique promotional taglines to photographs to customer's testimonials. The bottom line is the more information the search engine has regarding your business listing, the richer and more compelling the listing for the potential customer searching for you on the web. Add the use of specific keywords that connect customer searches to your search engine listing — subsequently to your Web site — and your listing could move to the top of the search listings; the higher your listing, the greater the chance that the customer will find you amongst your peers. This is the art and science of search engine optimization. It is essentially the proper alignment of every step in the search process with the landing page at your Web site.

Most search engines also provide you with the opportunity to advertise your business for a fee. The typical cost for the advertisement is based on a cost-per-click rate, meaning that you will only pay for clicks on your ad, and not simply for "impressions" or the times that your ad has been displayed on a search page. This means that it is not just important to write a very brief yet highly effective advertisement that will often bring the searcher to click on it but also to make sure you have developed a highly effective landing page with a great call-to-action so a customer's search doesn't end on the landing page without eliciting a positive action.

Web 2.0

Web 2.0 is associated with web-based applications that serve for interactive sharing of information and collaboration on the Internet. Social networking sites (Facebook, My Space, Twitter, etc.), video-sharing sites (youtube.com), and blogs are some of the more popular Web 2.0 vehicles commonly used in the fitness industry. These sites are primarily utilized as a tool to market a product, service, or business, or as a part of an integrated marketing strategy that uses public commentary via discussion boards or recorded and uploaded video to promote the service or product. Their widespread use and the ease with which the public can utilize these sites make them a great option as additional marketing modalities, not as primary vehicles, but as "supporting players" of sorts.

One way to look at it is that the primary objective online is to get potential customers to the business Web site landing page where it can prompt them to provide their e-mail address or other contact information in exchange for a free pass to the fitness facility, subscription to a free e-newsletter, or something that might be of interest to someone landing on the Web site. Acquiring this information puts the prospect into the sales funnel or tickler file — goal accomplished! Now, the objective is to maximize the number of visits to the Web site landing page. This is where Web 2.0 applications can help by providing an effective vehicle that funnels leads to the business landing page.

Social networking sites like Facebook or LinkedIn provide an opportunity to both build a business's relationship with customers and develop the business's brand. Facebook is a great business-to-customer interactive site, while LinkedIn serves as an effective business-to-business vehicle to do the same. Both also provide advertising tools allowing businesses to overtly promote their products and services. Such business-promoting ads work much like those made available by most search engines (such as Google), providing a cost-per-click charge instead of a traditional fee for placing the advertisement.

Facebook, in particular, with its more than 500 million users has fast become a mainstream tool used by nearly half of its users on a daily basis. This is powerful when used to market a business. The business creates a "profile" and then develops a "fan page" for the business. The interactive tools available are versatile, far-reaching, and easy to use; they will make it easy for the business to reach your customers regularly. All the business has to do is simply provide regular postings on its "wall" — its Facebook landing page — asking readers to comment on the postings. The more interactive the postings and fan page as a whole, the better. Ultimately, Facebook provides a ready-to-use tool to effectively communicate

	Jan				Feb				Mar				Apr				May				Jun			
Week	1	2	3	4	1	2	3	4	1	2	3	4	1	2	3	4	1	2	3	4	1	2	3	4
Events										▓														
Save the Date		▓																						
Register						▓																		
Reminder										▓														
Announcements																								
Product launch																								
Newsletter				▓				▓				▓				▓				▓				▓

	Jul				Aug				Sep				Oct				Nov				Dec			
Week	1	2	3	4	1	2	3	4	1	2	3	4	1	2	3	4	1	2	3	4	1	2	3	4
Events										▓														
Save the Date		▓																						
Register						▓																		
Reminder										▓														
Announcements																								
Product launch							▓																	
Newsletter				▓				▓				▓				▓				▓				▓

Figure 4-4. Master marketing schedule.

with current and prospective customers, building value and rapport with little time and effort as its primary investment.

E-Mail Marketing

E-mail marketing provides tremendous leverage at minimal cost. Its cost-effectiveness, however, depends on several things.

The business needs to set clear objectives prior to developing its e-mail marketing piece. Is it looking to develop leads and get inquiries from its list? Is it trying to convert contacts, present an offering, and close a sale? Is it simply building brand awareness or interacting with current customers? Its overall goal for the e-mail piece will determine its content, its frequency, and how to measure its success.

The e-mail distribution list must be comprised of contacts that have "opted in" or chosen to receive e-communications from the business. The business must understand current e-commerce law requirements, and how SPAM, Blocking, and Filtering might affect the successful delivery of the e-mail. For example, many e-mail service providers (*i.e.*, Gmail, Hotmail, etc.) automatically filter e-mails with the words "Free," "Guaranteed," "Credit Card" in the subject line or excessive punctuation in the body of the e-mail. The end result is that the contact never reads the e-mail, as it is diverted into their SPAM or Junk folder, or is blocked from delivery all together.

Ideally, the list should be comprised of contacts who have "explicitly" requested to be part of the mailing list. That is, they have proactively requested to be part of the list. Implicit permission, on the other hand, is when you include a contact because they happen to be a customer, or they have at some point agreed to receive a specific piece of information from you and end up on the list for future mailings. Most e-mail services (*i.e.*, Constant Contact, Vertical Response, etc.) provide simple-to-use tools that can be implemented when designing an e-mail that will prompt the contact to opt in and be explicitly added. They can also query the entire directory asking for their opt-in and as the positive responses come in, add that contact to the new list of confirmed contacts.

Learn about the contact's interests and use this information to segregate a general contacts list into topic-specific sublists. This way these subgroups can be targeted to send them only information that interests them. For example, a trainer who splits his or her time between working with adults, focusing on general fitness, and athlete conditioning for high school ballplayers can develop two separate e-mail pieces addressing the interests of these two diverse groups. This will likely increase the success of each e-mail being opened, read, and acted upon by the contacts.

Some more general things to do to enhance e-mail marketing include

- Use a "From" name that recipients will recognize. If the brand is more recognizable, use that in the "From" address. Avoid generic addresses (*i.e.*, sales@, info@).
- Personalize e-mails so that they speak directly to the recipient, addressing them by their first name.
- Create interest categories and prompt your contact to select their interests upon opting in.
- Instead of using a generic subject line (*i.e.*, "Monthly Newsletter") elect a subject that intrigues your recipient (*i.e.*, five foods that sabotage your weight loss efforts).

Figure 4-4 is a sample Master Schedule that can be used to lay out a marketing plan. The business should develop its Master Schedule along with its annual budget to ensure that the plan and the business overall are appropriately financed and to help plan out your staffing and operational activities throughout the year.

Determine message format and frequency. Make templates of e-mails so that they become visually familiar to recipients, and easy-to-develop future e-mails with a consistent look. Creating a Master Schedule will help coordinate the timing of each message for maximum impact (*i.e.*, newsletters on a monthly or quarterly basis, announce events or unique promos as needed). Track "opens" and "click-throughs" to identify when the recipient is most likely to read ("open") the message and respond to its offer ("click-through"). Generally, Tuesdays and Wednesdays between the hours of 10 am and 3 pm are best, but this may differ by business, industry, or client base. The bottom line is to track and test different days and times and go with what tends to work best (3).

The information provided in the body of the e-mail should be relevant and valuable to the reader. Here are some "rules of thumb" for e-mail marketing:

- Be clear and concise — Recipients will not spend a lot of time reading e-mails. Make it easy for them to read, by keeping it simple.
- Use appropriate graphics — Use only graphics that the business is legally entitled to use (royalty-free, or licensed for use). Do not use graphics that might be offensive to your recipients.
- Use white space effectively — Strategically placed banners and white space are useful in helping underlying messages stand out.
- Design for "above the fold" — Most often the top half or third of the first page of sent message will be visible in the preview screen of the recipient's inbox. This is known as the portion of the e-mail that is "above the fold." Make sure it includes a target message or "hook" to draw the recipient in and motivate them to read on.
- Include "Call to Action" links — The easier it is for the recipient to respond to the call to action, the better the success will be achieving the piece objective. If the goal is to build the list of prospects, provide a button the recipient can simply click to enter their request for more information. If the goal is to sell a product or service, the e-commerce shopping cart should be no more than a click away.
- Create sense of urgency — Providing a deadline or reason for the recipient to "act now" will increase your click-throughs.
- Capitalize and punctuate carefully — In fact, there is nothing more defeating than spelling and grammatical mistakes in e-mail copy. Get into the habit of routinely using a spell-check tool. If your e-mail service provider does not have one, use Word or another word processing application to develop e-mail text, spell-check it, and then copy and paste it into your e-mail template or simple e-mail program.
- Proofread over and over again — Ask a colleague to proofread your message and use their feedback to tweak the final edit.
- Remember to focus on content — It's not about the business. It's about what the business can do for the recipient. Be an expert.

Integrated Marketing

Technology continues to change the way the fitness industry plays the marketing game. Integrated marketing involves using a combination of e-marketing and/or hard copy direct mail advertising with a "personalized URL" (aka pURL). This strategy personalizes e-mail and hard copy pieces that are sent to the prospect urging the recipient to log on to "their" specially designed web-page, where the product or service offer is made. The technology makes it possible to individualize each marketing piece (*i.e.*, e-mail, postcard, and webpage) based on various demographic combinations that match up with the prospect. For example, the prospect's first name is used throughout each ad, as well as the Web site. Graphics in each piece also "speak to the prospect," depicting people, things, or activities that match up with the prospect's interests and life experience. If, for example, the prospect is a 50-year old white male living in the suburbs who loves to play golf, the ad might show an attractive, Caucasian, middle-aged male, next to his convertible, which is parked in front of his split-level home, with a golf-bag in the back seat. If the prospect is a 30-year-old African American male, who lives in an urban area, and plays golf, the ad could show a good-looking 30-ish African American male, hailing a cab on a city street with a golf bag hanging off his shoulder. Personalization increases the rate of response to most ads. This makes pURLs an effective approach to marketing fitness products and services.

YOU CAN'T QUALIFY WHAT YOU DON'T QUANTIFY

Smart marketing requires you to track the outcomes of your marketing. You must track and measure the success of each individual promotion, for each marketing medium. You keep those that provide you a consistent and worthwhile ROI, and discard those that don't elicit the response you are looking for. There are commonly accepted performance benchmarks (*i.e.*, 10% response for direct mail, 10% open-rate for e-mail marketing, video ads outperform nonvideo, etc.) (4), but it is important that you collect your own data and develop your own benchmarks. Every business is unique, as is each customer, and only by diligently tracking the outcomes of each marketing event will you come up with a consistently effective formula (5).

Some parameters that you should track for e-mail promotions include

- Number of e-mails sent — How many e-mail messages were sent?
- Bounced messages — How many e-mail messages were returned undeliverable?
- Delivery rate — Ratio of delivered messages versus sent messages.
- Opens — How many delivered messages were opened by the recipient?
- Clicks — How many recipients responded to the call to action in the message by clicking links?

- Forwards — How many delivered messages were forwarded to another recipient?
- Unsubscribes — How many recipients decided to opt out of future mailings?
- Spam complaints — How many recipients complained of receiving the e-mail as unsolicited?
- For direct mail campaigns, your tracking should include
- Number of pieces mailed — how many mailers were sent in a given campaign?
- Number of returns — how many mailers were returned undelivered?
- Number of queries sourced to mailer — how many leads were produced by a given mailer?

Regardless of the type of campaign, product, or service, ultimately the promotional pieces and marketing methods should be tied in to sales activities. For example, the business has budgeted 7 new member sales per week. If the overall sales closing percentage is 70%, then 10 sales opportunities per week will be needed in order to meet the budget. If all of marketing modalities combined yield a 1% return — that is, 1% of the total marketing hits become a sales opportunity — then it will be necessary to "tap" 1,000 leads through marketing in order to meet the sales opportunities budget number of 10 members/clients. This exercise makes it easy to budget and plan marketing activities. In this example, the sales closing percentage can be improved and the marketing's effectiveness can yield a higher return. Only by tracking all of these parameters over time will you master the ability to budget and "predict" marketing and sales outcomes effectively.

CHAPTER SUMMARY

Chapter 4 covered some of the more common marketing tactics used in the fitness business. It introduced the concepts of internal and external marketing, and highlighted conventional advertising as well as more "grassroots" types of guerilla marketing, providing sample display ads. It summarized some of the more common e-marketing strategies in the fitness industry and also tied in your marketing to your sales activities.

YOUR RESOURCES

Constant Contact — an e-mail service provider that has a robust coaching and support system. It is inexpensive and simple to use. For more information, go to: http://www.constantcontact.com

Vista Print — an online printing service for those sole proprietors who are on a tight budget. You can design your own business cards, brochures, and business letterhead. For more information, go to: http://www.vistaprint.com

ClubCom — a leader in the field of constructing and operating private television networks for targeted communal audiences. It is a commonly used medium for in-house marketing in fitness facilities. For more information, go to: www.ClubCom.com

Exercise is Medicine — a joint effort by ACSM and the American Medical Association that envisions making physical activity and exercise a standard part of a disease prevention and treatment medical paradigm in the United States. One of its primary objectives is to bridge the gap between medical physicians and health and fitness professionals. For more information, go to: http://www.exerciseismedicine.org/index.htm

REFERENCES

1. Merriam-Webster, Inc. 2011. Available at: http://www.merriam-webster.com/dictionary/marketing
2. American College of Sports Medicine. *ACSM's Resources for the Personal Trainer*. 2nd ed. Baltimore (MD): Lippincott, Williams, & Wilkins, 2007.
3. Constant Contact. *E-mail Marketing Workbook*. 2nd ed. Constant Contact; Waltham (MA), 2008.
4. Google, Inc. Whitepaper: DoubleClick for Advertisers, U.S. advertisers, a cross section of major ad sizes only, January – December 2009. DoubleClick by Google, Mountain View, (CA). 2010. [Internet]. [cited 2011 August 21]. Available from: www.google.com/en/us/doubleclick/pdfs/DoubleClick-07-2010-DoubleClick-Benchmarks-Report-2009-Year-in-Review-US.pdf.
5. Constant Contact. *Best Practices in E-mail Marketing*. Constant Contact; Waltham (MA), 2008.

5 Service

Chapter Objectives

After reading this chapter, the reader will:

- Understand the importance of professional service delivery in providing the member with an optimal service experience
- Understand that some of the most basic customer service skills include approachability, professional appearance, good communication skills, and an in-depth understanding of the company's mission and policies
- Understand that the key to effective customer service is meeting the health club member's expectations

THE HOSPITALITY PARADIGM

The fitness industry is part of the service business sector. For most fitness professionals, it is easy to see how they are indeed in a "service business." Good customer service helps keep current customers as well as attract new ones. Before we take a closer look at customer service, we need to understand a very basic premise. Customers don't purchase service. They purchase experiences. The goal in developing a business's customer service system is to provide its members with extraordinary experiences.

In Part 2, we discuss developing a business vision, progressing through the exercise of writing its mission and value statements. These two set the stage for management and staff, providing a guide or paradigm that clearly defines "how" they do their job while delivering their products and services.

There are some basic skills and personality attributes that go a long way in delivering optimal levels of customer service. These are traits that every employee should have. It is important to look for these traits when hiring employees and then train and educate staff to make sure that they are thoroughly equipped to deliver on customers' expectations.

Approachability

Members, guests, and clients should always feel welcome. Frontline staff should exude warmth and be approachable. A smile is something that should always be part of their repertoire. A smile makes members feel welcome. Here are some simple guidelines that will ensure that you are always approachable.

- When a member approaches you:
  - Stand before a member approaches you (or is 10 feet away).
  - Make eye contact.
  - Smile.
  - Greet the member warmly within 5 feet: "Hello; welcome; may I assist you; how are you today?" (This is often described as the 10-foot/5-foot rule in hospitality training).
  - Use open body language — hands out of pocket, arms uncrossed.
  - Thank the guest.
- When passing a member in or around the facility:
  - Make eye contact as you are about to pass the guest within 10 feet.
  - Smile.
  - Greet the guest warmly within 5 feet: "Hello; how is your workout? how are you today?"
  - Use open body language — hands out of pocket, arms uncrossed.
- Make a great first impression — Always display a professional appearance:
  - Wear your complete uniform with name tag, if applicable.
  - Adhere to proper grooming and hygiene.
  - Smile.
  - Display open, receptive body language.
  - Show good posture at all times.
  - Provide your full, undivided attention whenever with a member.
- Provide professional and warm verbal communication:
  - Use terms like "Good morning"; "Good afternoon."
  - Always say "Thank you" as the member departs.

- Ask the member "How do you feel?" after a workout, class, etc.
- Show genuine interest in the guest and say things like "It's great to see you..."

Appearance

The guidelines listed below provide a general example that would be appropriate in most fitness facilities. Keep in mind that specific guidelines are going to differ from facility to facility, but, in general, following such guidelines may not "help" interaction with the member, but it will certainly not "hurt" the member's perception. Following the suggested guidelines will increase the chances of meeting the member's expectations and reduce the risk of making a "wrong impression."

- Uniforms: When applicable, team members should wear and handle their uniform with care so that it remains in good condition at all times. Uniforms must be clean and neatly pressed with shirts tucked into pants or shorts. A complete uniform must be worn at all times while working.
- Shoes: Should be appropriate and safe to your work area. Sneakers should be clean and in good condition.
- Perfume/deodorant: Due to close contact with members, use of deodorants or antiperspirant is absolutely required; however, heavy perfumes or colognes are discouraged.
- Earrings: For women, simple earrings, one in each ear, are permissible (employees should check with their supervisor prior to wearing earrings to work). For safety reasons, long dangling earrings or large hoops should not be worn. Men may not wear earrings to work.
- Facial jewelry: No nose rings or any other facial jewelry are to be worn by either men or women.
- Hair: Employees' hair must be clean and neatly combed at all times. Colored streaks, tails, or sculpturing are not permitted. Hats and caps are not permitted, unless part of the uniform. For men, the length of the employee's hair should not exceed his shirt collar. Beards or mustaches may be permissible, but must be neat and well trimmed (employees should check with their supervisor before reporting to work with a beard or mustache).
- Other: Gum chewing is not allowed in the fitness area or by any staff responsible for answering the telephone. Employees should not be eating or drinking in any area that is not designated for eating or drinking.

Clothing that is not permitted for all employees may include jeans of any color or length, t-shirts, ripped or worn clothing, cropped shirts, beach sandals, scuffed or dirty footwear, uncovered jog bras, or other unprofessional attire. Employees are expected to utilize sound judgment in preparing themselves to report for work.

Knowledgeable

Employees who have a clear understanding of your services, policies, and procedures, and who also understand and "live your mission" will be your best customer service providers. They are able to answer your customers' questions quickly, clearly, and completely, and are often empowered to present solutions to customer concerns.

Communication

It is often said that the best salespeople are not the best talkers, but instead the best listeners. Good listening skills are invaluable not just in selling but also in day-to-day interactions. Verbal communication should always be clear and appropriate. Use of slang and profanity are obvious no-nos. Tone of voice should be pleasant and friendly. Your best communicators will consistently listen to the customer, ensure that they understand the specific concerns raised by the customer, and respond in an effective manner. Figure 5-1 provides a "good-listener's checklist" with effective listening behaviors for the good communicator.

Communicating by telephone presents a challenge, because you and your customer lose the visual input that you would have when speaking in person. You must try to "paint a picture" for the member when speaking by phone (Fig. 5-2).

Effective telephone communication checklist

- Put a smile in your voice.
- Answer the phone under three rings.
- Use an appropriate scripted greeting, introduce your facility, yourself, and offer to be of assistance.

Good Listener's Checklist

☐ Look at the speaker; observe body language and pick up subtle nuances in speech

☐ Ask questions

☐ Summarize frequently, repeating in their own words what was said (this checks understanding and gives feedback)

☐ Give speakers time to articulate their thoughts

☐ Remain poised, calm and emotionally controlled

☐ Respond by nodding and with affirmative language

☐ Look alert and interested

☐ Let people finish what they are saying before giving your opinion

☐ Check their understanding by repeating the other's point of view before disagreeing

---

Figure 5-1. The good listener's checklist — practicing these listening behaviors will enhance communication with customers.

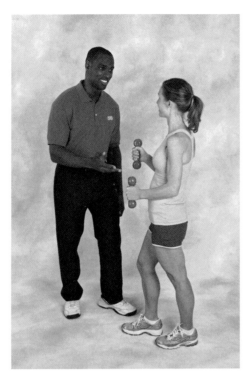

Figure 5-2. Personal trainer communicating effectively with a client upon the completion of an exercise. Reprinted with permission from ACSM's Resources for the Personal Trainer. 3rd ed. Philadelphia (PA): Lippincott Williams & Wilkins, 2010.

- Ask the caller for their name, and use their name throughout the call.
- Be prepared with pen and paper to take information, if necessary.
- Listen actively.
- Don't get defensive; empathize with the caller's situation.
- Know proper on-hold technique (caller should never be left on hold for longer than 30 seconds), and how to conference or take message.
- Confirm information and, if necessary, how you can help; make sure the caller has clear expectations and call outcome.
- Thank them and wait for them to hang up first.

E-mail technology can be a blessing when used effectively, but can also open up a can of worms, when used ineffectively. Remember that tone is not easily conveyed via e-mail. This means that messages that are not clear and direct may be misconstrued and misunderstood.

E-mail communication checklist

- Be concise and to the point.
- Avoid provocative/angry language.

- Give much thought to sending unsolicited e-mail, and make sure that there is value to the recipient. If you don't, they may very well consider it junk mail and delete it unread.
- Keep attachments to a minimum.
- CC when someone needs to know the information but no response is necessary. BCC when sending to a large group of people or when you do not want to disclose the recipients.
- Check spelling and punctuation before sending.
- Include information in the subject line. If your e-mail requires immediate attention, your subject line can convey this urgency.
- Respond within 24 hours, when you receive an e-mail.
- Program your e-mail account if you aren't checking messages for an extended period of time. Provide an auto-response out-of-office message that clearly communicates when you will respond to e-mail messages and provides an alternative point of contact, again managing their expectations.

Problem-Solving Skills

A key portion of effective customer service involves resolving customer issues. You must be able to analyze information, identify the issue, and resolve the situation in a timely fashion. For many frontline employees, this requires making quick and accurate decisions. Good problem solvers know how to utilize their resources to obtain information and are able to effectively prioritize their time, and respond effectively and professionally to customers' concerns.

Dealing with upset customers checklist

- Listen: Take them aside and let them vent, and use active listening skills (repeat the complaint, ask questions, take notes when appropriate).
- Empathize: Show care and concern, but do not complain yourself. Use effective language ("I would be upset too...").
- Apologize: Be sincere, know what you're apologizing for, and treat each customer with respect throughout the interaction.
- Take ownership and take action: Thank the member and tell them what you can do (specifically), find a solution you both agree on, and proactively follow up (call, e-mail, next time you see them, slip a note in their locker).

After the member leaves:

- Reflect on what happened — what went well, what could have been done differently?
- Don't take it personally.

- Don't talk about it unless it's a lesson that will help coworkers, or ask what they would do.
- Record what happened in the "Daily Log" or other communication tool for the team.
- Communicate what happened with management to correct procedures and prevent future problems.
- Fix the issue so it doesn't happen again.

Action-Oriented Task Manager

Customer service often involves completing several tasks simultaneously. Most customer service responsibilities include daily goals and deadlines that must be met. Good customer service skills include the ability to meet these goals in a timely fashion. Employees must be action-oriented and take ownership, manage their time wisely, and work effectively both independently and in a team environment.

Professionalism

Professionalism is an integral part of customer interaction. Customer service representatives represent their company and their products to the public. You must be respectful, courteous, and demonstrate confidence in your company and its products.

"Gym Etiquette" — General Rules of Professional Conduct for Fitness Professionals

On and Around the Fitness Floor

- Focus on the member at all times.
- Provide constant feedback, give them positive encouragement and spot when necessary.
- Proper body language is extremely important. Do not sit or lean on a piece of equipment while the member is working out.
- Aside from the safety factor, if the member perceives that you are disinterested and not caring, the quality of their workout will be compromised.
- Help keep the facility in order and presentable.
  - Put back equipment.
  - Make periodic checks of the changing rooms and locker room facilities and make sure they are clean.
  - Let the members know where everything is: the phone system, the emergency alarm, equipment, office, etc.

The Personal Training Client's Program

- Update personal training client's program as soon as any change in their condition occurs.
- When in doubt, consult with trainer's manual or management regarding special populations.
- The more closely you monitor your client's variations in structural and metabolic conditions, the safer the program will be.
- Have a sincere commitment to provide the highest-quality program.
- Provide safe, effective, and efficient instruction and provide members a great experience.
- Listen closely to what the member says, especially as it relates to pain. Don't assume you know their pain threshold, or how the exercise feels to them.

During the Training Session or Group Exercise Class

- Approach each member with an open mind; don't make judgments or discriminate based on appearances.
- Treat each member with courtesy and respect.
- Treat members equally in your time and attention, but according to the individual's needs. For example, provide exercise guidance or modifications for less experienced participants.
- Choose words carefully in order not to offend.
- Provide a safe and comfortable environment that engenders trust and mutual respect.
- Keep business relationships on a professional level. (Do not give out personal information such as telephone numbers, address, etc.)
- Maintain clear and honest communications.
- Dress in a professional manner as outlined by management's grooming standards.
- Enhance the fitness industry image.
- Refuse any gifts that are intended to influence a decision and are purely for personal gain. (*This does not include gratuities rendered for services.*)
- Do not make false claims regarding the potential benefits of the services rendered.
- Uphold and enhance public appreciation and trust for the health and fitness industries, and help eliminate prejudices in the profession.
- Comply with all applicable business, employment, and copyright laws. Cite all sources used when writing an article, or using information that is not your own.

Setting Training Standards

The personal training manager is ultimately responsible for the safety and customer satisfaction of every personal training client. Therefore, it is necessary that standards are set for delivering personal training services in a manner that is consistent with industry standards for safety and that will insure excellent customer service that is consistently delivered. Here are some guidelines for setting the department's service standards (1):

- Trainers must give their undivided attention to their clients. This means that trainers are watching clients at all times and spotting exercises with appropriate techniques. Policy parameters should be specific. Talking on cell phones, talking with other trainers or other members, and watching TV monitors are examples of unacceptable behaviors that would not meet training standards. In addition, if a trainer spends much of the training session talking about his/her personal affairs, it will be difficult for the trainer to fully focus on the client's workout and exercise technique.
- Trainers must show up for training sessions on time and end training sessions on time. Trainers must respect the training client's time and schedule.
- There should be a dress standard for the department's personal trainers. If possible, trainers should wear a shirt with a facility logo and the words "Personal Trainer." The shirt, along with established standards for pants and shoes, will insure a professional look for the training department, while providing training department advertising to other members.
- Trainers should document and write down every client's workout, as well as any measurements, tests, and performance tracking for that client. The training department manager should provide a standardized training card for the trainers' use. There should be a designated training file where the training cards are kept that is accessible to both the training client and other trainers. If a client wants to work out without the trainer, or another trainer needs to cover a training session because of trainer illness, vacation, etc., the training cards are readily available.
- A client confidentiality policy should be maintained. Trainers should be reminded that they should never discuss any client's personal information with other trainers or clients. Trainers must respect their clients' privacy and be trustworthy.
- Trainer honesty and scope of practice standards should be emphasized. If a trainer does not know the answer to a client's health- or fitness-related questions, the trainer needs to admit that he or she does not have that information. The trainer can volunteer to research the topic and provide an answer at the next training session. If the client is asking for medical advice

or a diagnosis, the trainer must not overstep his or her scope of practice, but should explain that the client needs to consult a physician for that information.

- Personal trainers must maintain personal training certifications, cardio-pulmonary resuscitation certification, and liability insurance, if it is not provided by the fitness facility. Records of trainer certification and professional liability insurance should be kept in their employee files.
- Look at the speaker; observe body language and pick up subtle nuances in speech.
- Ask questions.
- Summarize frequently, repeating in their own words what was said (this checks understanding and gives feedback).
- Give speakers time to articulate their thoughts.
- Remain poised, calm, and emotionally controlled.
- Respond by nodding and with affirmative language.
- Look alert and interested.
- Let people finish what they are saying before giving your opinion.
- Check their understanding by repeating the other's point of view.

CHAPTER SUMMARY

The fitness industry is a service business whose success is dependent on providing its customers with optimal service experiences. In order to deliver this optimal service, staff should be carefully selected at point of hire and thoroughly trained thereafter to be properly equipped to respond to members' needs and situations. The most basic customer service skills include approachability, professional appearance, good communication skills, and an in-depth understanding of the company's mission and policies. Personal trainers and group exercise instructors should project a proactive professional demeanor that sheds a positive light upon them, their club, their profession, and the industry.

YOUR RESOURCES

IHRSA's Resource Center
http://www.IHRSA.org
Club Industry's Step-by-Step column is a great resource, featuring many articles on Customer Service and Member Retention, as well as Personal Training and Management.
http://clubindustry.com/
Entertainment Cruises, Our Service System [Internet]
http://www.entertainmentcruises.com/entertainment-cruises/our-service-system

The Ritz-Carlton Hotel Company, L.L.C. — "Gold Standards", Careers, The Ritz-Carlton Hotel Company, L.L.C., 2011 as seen at: ***http://corporate.ritzcarlton.com/en/About/Gold-Standards.htm***

Dale Carnegie's Golden Book. Dale Carnegie Training. [Internet] Dale Carnegie and Associates, Inc. 2006.
www.dalecarnegie.com

Fitness Management magazine (recently merged with *Athletic Business* magazine) is a good resource for articles on club management and service.
http://www.athleticbusiness.com/fitnessmanagement

REFERENCES

1. American College of Sports Medicine. *ACSM's Resources for the Personal Trainer.* 2nd ed. Baltimore (MD): Lippincott, Williams, & Wilkins, 2007. p.474

Operations, Administration, and Management

Chapter Objectives

After reading this chapter, the reader will:

- Understand that effective program administration creates safe, successful programs and services and reduces the risk of problems and legal situations

- Understand that the program manager ensures that the program meets the often-changing standards and practices for fitness facilities and services

- Understand that the program manager needs to have a basic knowledge of management and financial principles

- Understand that the program manager must coordinate many interrelated components and services

- Understand that the input of the facility's upper management (*e.g.*, the facility owner, the fitness center's general manager) into program development and implementation is crucial and must be solicited by the program director/manager

THE ROAD LESS TRAVELED: CAREER GROWTH INTO ADMINISTRATION AND MANAGEMENT

It is smart for businesses to cross-train their employees so that they are capable of filling multiple roles in various departments. Many frontline fitness professionals become highly skilled and proficient not just in the technical aspects of their job but also in dealing with the operational challenges faced daily throughout their facility. Management strives to be "lean and mean," running their business as efficiently as possible. It typically looks to grow its organization from within, and developing "homegrown" leaders is a great way of maximizing a business's resources and developing future managers. There is nothing more gratifying than managing the growth of frontline workers throughout their tenure at a fitness center and experiencing their enthusiasm and initiative to branch out, learn, and ultimately lead.

Wearing the management hat forces employees to shift their perspective and begin to work "on" their business, as opposed to "in" their business. The smooth running and overall success of the business become the primary objectives in the employee's mind. From budgeting, to maintenance, to hiring and firing, the fitness professional learns to touch every aspect of the business.

Characteristics of a Good Program Director/Manager

Keeping in mind that a fitness professional's career will typically go through a "stepping stone" process, going from fitness instructor, to fitness director, to assistant manager, and then perhaps to general manager, and understanding that depending on the work environment these job titles might be interchangeable, let's look at the various responsibilities that the fitness professional will tackle as he or she goes from the frontlines to the back office.

A program director or manager designs and monitors the delivery of exercise programs. This includes organizing the required resources, arranging the program and staffing schedules, guiding the staff or clients through the program, and purchasing equipment and supplies. On the "backend," the program manager must also assess program and client outcomes and needs. The manager must first establish goals for the program. Then by monitoring program outcomes and facility safety, many aspects of the program can be accurately evaluated, so that any changes warranted by the evaluation can be implemented.

The program manager must demonstrate good communication skills providing leadership, and developing and motivating both staff and clients, coordinating staff and program development, and evaluating staff and programs. The program manager must possess strong teaching and coaching skills, providing education and training for staff. Developing and implementing a staff training program and soliciting feedback from staff and clients help the manager deliver training and education that are relevant and enhance employees' ability to deliver service as envisioned by management.

The program manager must possess the ability to promote programs, by understanding the benefits of the program, communicating those benefits to staff and clients, and encouraging participation.

Basic Responsibilities of a Program Manager

Given the ideal characteristics and core competencies listed above, there are some common responsibilities shared by most program managers. Ultimately, the primary goal of a program manager is the development and success of the program. To this end, a program manager must assess client interest and satisfaction through program observation, surveys and focus groups, and client and staff feedback.

A program manager observes all aspects of the program, including

- Staff performance
- Efficiency of facility design and layout
- Efficiency of programs and services
- Cleanliness and environmental condition of the facility

A program manager implements policies and procedures, including

- Assisting staff in understanding and enforcing all rules and policies
- Communicating emergency procedures clearly
- Confirming understanding in the day-to-day operations of the facility

A program manager determines availability of resources, including

- Equipment
- Supplies
- Space
- Staff

A program manager manages the program's and/or facility's financials, including

- Budget of costs and expected revenues
- Cost/benefit analyses of specific programs
- Containing costs within budgetary limits
- Ensuring that program margins are in line with profitability goals

A program manager promotes the program through marketing efforts, and designs promotions that attract participants.

A program manager schedules programs appropriately, taking into account

- Target audience
- Staff availability and strengths/weaknesses
- Other programs

A program manager manages emergency preparedness. He or she

- Ensures that staff is well-versed in all facility emergency protocols
- Ensures that all safety equipment (*e.g.*, automated external defibrillator, AED) is in operating order
- Schedules and periodically administers emergency drills

A program manager evaluates and appraises staff performance. He or she

- Ensures full disclosure of staff expectations and responsibilities
- Ensures effective delivery of all pertinent training and education so that staff is capable of effectively doing their job
- Conducts counseling sessions whenever necessary in a fair and timely fashion to correct staff behaviors

Wearing the Human Resources Hat

In a business where member retention and referrals are dependent on customer satisfaction, recruiting and hiring candidates with the right personality traits and skill sets is crucial. But even the most talented personnel require comprehensive training and continued development to ensure that they can deliver on the company's mission and service promise.

One of the most important areas of focus in a typical fitness facility is ensuring the optimal staffing of the facility. In its simplest terms, fitness facilities offer space with equipment, some level of programming, and staff to deliver it all to the customer. Once the facility is open and most capital expenses (start-up costs) have been spent, payroll will account for the biggest percentage of a facility's operational expenses. It is easy to see why optimal staffing is crucial to the success of any fitness business, and management's role in recruiting, hiring, training, and developing that staff is paramount.

"Only the Friendly Need Apply"

It is imperative when hiring all employees that the focus is on hiring "people who love people." Employees should love to be around people. They should posses the heart of a servant. If a prospective employee comes in for an interview and does not smile and exude warmth during the interview, what would ever make you think that they'll start smiling once they're hired? Remember that so long as the prospective employee possesses the credentials and education required for the position, management will likely be able to train and provide them the technical skills they will need for the job. Management will not, however, be able to provide them with a personality through technical training. If smiling does not come naturally, it won't come at all, and moving on to the next candidate is the safest bet.

Why is smiling so important? Fitness centers are an intimidating place for most "civilians." While fitness professionals feel right at home in a health club, between the massive "spaceship-like" equipment, and the svelte, bikini-ready bodies (real or perceived), most would-be members are too scared to even consider walking into a health club, let alone feeling comfortable participating in the club on a regular basis. The entire staff should have one primary job in mind, and that is to SMILE and provide a welcoming environment for all guests and members. Once the interviewee has passed the "smile test," position-specific requirements and role-playing scenarios should be presented.

Hiring Technical Staff — Personal Trainers and Group Exercise Instructors

The following are important steps to follow when hiring personal trainers, group exercise instructors, and any other "technical staff" (*i.e.*, massage therapists, estheticians, etc.):

- Resumes should be reviewed carefully for educational background, current certifications, recent training experience with a variety of clientele, and innovative training programs.
- When contacting applicants for interviews, they should be asked to bring copies of their current fitness and CPR-AED/First Aid certifications to the interview appointment. In states where professional licensing is required (*i.e.*, massage therapists), interviewees must present current copies of these documents at the time of their interview. This may prevent an undesired realization after hiring that the employee's credentials have expired.
- The manager should create a list of questions to ask all applicants. The questions should be practical, including scenarios specific to the scope of practice for the prospective employee. These could include real-world scenarios that will require
  - The trainer to discuss training program options for hypothetical "special-pops" clients
  - The group exercise instructor to provide exercise modifications for class participants
  - The massage therapist to provide a pretreatment screening for high-risk clients

- The applicant's availability and scheduling preference for work-shifts and appointments should be clearly assessed and agreed to at the time of the interview, prior to a job offer. If the department needs an evening trainer, and the interviewee is already training elsewhere in the evening, the trainer/manager needs to know that information to effectively plan for staffing needs.

- A practical or "hands-on" component should be part of the interview process. The prospective employee should demonstrate his or her skills and abilities as he or she pertains to the proposed job (*i.e.*, exercises and spotting techniques for a prospective personal trainer, sample group class for a prospective group exercise instructor, 30-minute massage for a prospective massage therapist, etc.). It is imperative that the manager or other employee(s) be designated to play the role(s) of hypothetical clients and provide the manager with pertinent feedback to assess how the prospect performed and interacted with them. Never allow a prospective employee to "demonstrate" their skills on actual clients. This can present very serious liability implications and is never worth the risk of either hurting a client or angering a client due to an interviewee's "poor audition."

Job Descriptions

- Each staff position needs a specific, written job description that clearly details the duties, responsibilities, and evaluation criteria for the position.
- The job descriptions for all positions in the organization should be part of the policies and procedures (P&P) manual.
- An effective job description is tailored to the specific needs and goals of the individual program.
- Because all possible duties and responsibilities cannot be detailed, some degree of flexibility and adaptability must be built into each job description.
- The job descriptions may be used to highlight preferred behaviors during employee counseling sessions along with the P&P Manual.
- The job description also provides criteria to evaluate during the employee performance review.

Once Hired

It is important that employees know from day one what management's expectations are, as well as what they should expect from management. Job responsibilities should be clearly defined and discussed by the employees and their direct report(s) as part of the final interview process. Once hired, basic employment policies should be clearly outlined and reviewed as part of the payroll forms ritual. Just because these policies are outlined clearly in a P&P Manual, "don't expect what you don't inspect." Review such policies directly with the new employee. These policies (*i.e.*, uniform and grooming requirements, paid leave policies and procedures, payroll and employee benefits procedures, etc.) may be delivered either by a human resources representative or general management.

Initial staff training should include a general orientation. This session is designed to help employees understand the "lay of the land" and begin to identify with the company. This progressive indoctrination will teach employees about the company they are now part of. This is where their importance to the success of the business begins to take shape. This general orientation should include

- The organization's mission statement and service promise, which provides the paradigm with which the employee can make effective day-to-day decisions.
- The organizational structure of the company (who the players are, how the departments are structured, and how they interrelate with the employee's department).
- A company snapshot — where it "lives" in the industry, how it has developed into a business, and what the current big-picture company goals are.
- General employee policies and procedures (many of which have already been discussed in prior training) should be repeated to ensure that they are understood — note that adoption of company philosophy is an ongoing process.
- How to be a productive employee.

After setting the tone with a company orientation, the employee should go through an in-depth departmental training that addresses how it relates to overall company goals. This training should include

- The department's goals and service objectives, which clearly relate to the employee's specific job tasks, while maintaining departmental customer service objectives.
- The organizational structure of the department, the chain of command, day-to-day resources, and how to best communicate with management and other employees.
- A snapshot of the department and what it provides for the company and customers, as well as the current goals of the department.
- Specific departmental policies and procedures.
- Employee's and direct report's expectations.
- How to be a productive team member.

Next, the employee should receive job-specific task training. This is where day-to-day technical tasks are covered. It should provide a comprehensive step-by-step learning opportunity that will give the employee the specific tools for their daily job tasks. This may include

- Opening/closing/operational procedures (those applicable). It is important to keep in mind that cross-training employees across departments is a good thing.
- Systems (software/equipment) training (member database and check-in, telephone/intercom system operation, training equipment, etc.).
- Technical service training (fitness assessment and exercise programming guidelines for trainers, postworkout shake recipes or procedures for juice bar personnel, membership service criteria for reception staff, etc.).
- Emergency procedures.

Now it's time to shift focus to the employee's ongoing professional development. Continuing education is required for all employees. Beyond the typical trainers' technical training (writing business memos, professional communication skills, customer service, management skills), health club owners and management can decide on the type of education and if it is most feasible to provide continuing education in-house or off premises. Companies can provide an incentive and subsidize approved educational experiences. Such expenses should be put in the operational budget during its planning stage for the fiscal year.

Staff Competency and Development

Maintaining staff competency is a major responsibility of the program manager.

- Continuous professional development is important for staff competency.
  - The program director/manager must guide staff in seeking out opportunities for professional development.
- A typical staff is multidisciplinary. The various staff members will have varying needs and opportunities for professional development. This may include
  - Exercise physiologists
  - Personal trainers
  - Group exercise instructors
  - "Specialists" — yoga and/or Pilates instructors, strength and conditioning specialists
  - Massage therapists
- Staff meetings focused on professional development issues that can be aimed at a particular group of staff (*i.e.*, operation of a new exercise machine) or that can encompass the entire staff (*i.e.*, customer service issues).
- In-service staff meetings are an excellent forum for professional development. In-services can utilize staff skills or the knowledge and skills from outside professionals.

- Encouraging staff to seek outside professional development will greatly enhance the skills and abilities of all staff members. Opportunities may include: Continuing Education Credit/Continuing Education Unit-approved continuing education sessions, attending professional conferences, seeking additional certifications.
- Good communication among staff members is an essential component of overall staff competency. Strategies to foster staff communication include
  - Following lines of communication depicted on the program's organizational flowchart
  - Holding regular staff meetings, both formal and informal, with the entire staff as well as with selected staff members involved in a particular program, project, or issue
  - Ensuring that communication works in both directions, thus creating an "open-door" policy
- Certification and licensure of various staff members is another aspect of staff competency.
  - Credentialing is relatively standardized for some staff (*e.g.*, registered dietitians) but is less so for other positions (*e.g.*, exercise physiologists).
  - It is accepted that certified staff are more likely to be consistent in their care and training and to possess a greater level of knowledge and abilities.
  - The health/fitness manager must be aware that many fitness certifications exist and that some do not follow the higher standards that organizations like the ACSM believe are necessary for safe and effective care of fitness clients. Understanding which certifications are acceptable is an important part of being a health/fitness manager.

Keep in mind that the training process is ongoing. An employee will not live the mission statement unless he or she lives it each and every day. It takes time for an employee to learn the skills, adopt the corporate philosophy, and finally make it their own. Creating a checklist of developmental objectives that is kept in an employee's personnel file will ease the annual employee performance evaluation process and identify where an employee can enhance their work skills through training to increase their value to the company. Managers, who make it their responsibility to provide the tools and learning environment that will enhance their employees' performance, will retain and develop employees over the long haul — ensuring their employees' success, as well as that of their business.

Profit and Loss for Fitness Professionals

It is rare to find fitness professionals who are as comfortable analyzing profit-loss statements as they are assessing VO_2. The truth is that the most important take-home for any fitness manager is to understand their budgets and projections, so that they can effectively manage their business on a day-to-day basis.

Part 2 of this book will provide a step-by-step development process and in-depth look at budgets. What is a budget? In its most practical terms, an expense budget provides a line-by-line breakdown of running the business costs, and an income budget provides a line-by-line breakdown of projected income expected over a specific time frame from business activities. A manager's goal is to stay as close to the planned budget numbers as possible, and manage the day-to-day operations of the facility to keep the numbers in line. Specifically, if you are behind on sales projections, you need to drum up some business to accelerate cash flow into the business and bring income projections back in line. If you are ahead on the expense side, you need to tighten the purse strings and control spending until it is back in line. Of course, one can compensate for the other, so keep an eye on both money coming in and money going out. If expenses are up because sales commissions are up, chances are that sales income is also up beyond prior expectations, and should compensate for the increased expense.

Fitness Professional as Jack of All Trades

A fitness center tends to provide plenty of opportunities for "operational chaos." In other words, you have a lot of moving parts — members, equipment, showers, light fixtures, etc. They all need a little special attention every now and then. The trick is to stay on top of maintenance and repair issues. This will prevent simple situations from becoming operational chaos.

It is a good idea to keep a running record of all equipment, especially those pieces that might require significant maintenance (*i.e.*, treadmills). Keep these records in a three-ring binder. Create a single record sheet for each piece of equipment, making sure to include the vendor's name and contact information, date of purchase, warantee expiration date (if any), model number, serial number, and any identifying code used on the equipment in the facility. Many clubs number each unit so that it is easily identifyable by members and staff alike. Whenever there is an incident on any piece of equipment, it is recorded on its asigned record sheet. For example, (when it happened) date, (what happened) cable snapped, (what was done) called Richie at ABC cardio for repair, (outcome) repair visit pending. This process seems tedious, but will prevent a lot of heartache later, and can even help demonstrate proactive maintenance (*i.e.*, scheduled flipping of treadmill decks or changing belts) if an injury occurs on a given piece of equipment. This may support the business' defense in a liability case.

Another operational nightmare for some clubs that don't plan properly is inventory. It is important to keep accurate records of both wholesale/retail items, as well as amenities (*i.e.*, paper towels, shower gel), and product/program items (*i.e.*, juice bar fruit or protein powder for smoothies and shakes). The better handle you have on the quantity and their frequency of purchase, the more budgetary control you will have over these areas. Not to mention the fact that at some point, it all falls to bottom line.

CHAPTER SUMMARY

Many fitness professionals live for their love of helping others and positively changing lives through fitness. There are a few that step out of their comfort zone to learn and thrive in leadership roles in a fitness facility. Many take on responsibilities including staff and program management and development, day-to-day operations, and finally budgetary management and oversite. It is important as one travels this path to realize that even though you are in some ways distancing yourself from that which you love — actually touching and impacting your clients — you may actually exponentially enhance your reach through management, touching more clients than you ever could on your own. The effective manager is a strong leader and effective mentor, as well as a creative program developer. It is in wearing these hats that a manager can pass along his or her "gifts" to the staff so that they can go out and touch the masses.

REFERENCES

1. American College of Sports Medicine. *ACSM's Resources for the Personal Trainer.* 2nd ed. Baltimore (MD): Lippincott, Williams, & Wilkins, 2007.
2. *American College of Sports Medicine, Program and Administration/Management, in ACSM's Certification Review.* Baltimore (MD): Lippincott, Williams, & Wilkins, 2010. p. 197–208.
3. Pire, N. Developing and retaining a professional staff, step by step column in ClubIndustry.com, 2006. [Internet]. [cited 2011 August 21]; Penton Media, Inc. Available from: http://clubindustry.com/stepbystep/clubs/retaining-professional-staff/

7 Business Policy Development and Risk Management

Chapter Objectives

After reading this chapter, the reader will:

- Understand the importance of developing a mission and vision for their business
- Define core values that provide guiding paradigms to follow as business policies and procedures are developed and as employees carry them out on a day-to-day basis
- Understand the importance of providing tools and training for employees so that they routinely use the company's mission, vision, and core values statements to guide their behaviors at work
- Recognize professional standards and the Code of Ethics for ACSM-certified and registered professionals
- Recognize the most common potential areas of professional liability
- Understand the basics of risk management

DEVELOPING BUSINESS POLICIES THAT WORK

When launching a business, the fitness professional must wear many hats. Your focus shifts back and forth from fitness programming to financial considerations, to customer service and liability issues. Legal and financial implications related to the delivery of your core fitness services are crucial to your success and often dictate what you include in your business policies and standard operating procedures. Not paying attention to these details may bring an otherwise successful business crashing down. When assessing the many aspects of your business, you will find a list of things you will want to do, and another list of things that you want to make sure you don't do. Developing business policies that help guide you, your employees, and your customers will help keep your business on track, optimizing service delivery and minimizing liability risks.

Mission, Vision, and Values — A Guiding Light for Your Business

Business policies should be designed around a set paradigm or philosophy. The paradigm may be defined by the organization's mission, vision, and value statements. A company's mission statement describes "what" it is in business to do. For example, "XYZ, Inc. strives to maximize shareholder value by growing its customer base, increasing the income per customer visit, and retaining its customers over the long haul." This mission statement clearly defines its primary goal as increasing per share value to its owners or shareholders. It also lists the three primary business activities as finding new customers, selling more products and services to its customers, and keeping those customers, or maintaining market share, for an extended period of time.

A vision statement describes the company's impact on its customers or community, and what it sees in the company's future. A facility that features a fitness and recreational program for teens might envision a "no teens left behind" mentality with a vision statement like, "A program for every teen in our community."

A value statement or a company's "core values" are clearly stated principles that define universal expectations and preferred modes of behavior in an organization. A core values statement serves as a "how-to" guide for daily work activities. If "excellence in service" is one of your business's core values, set policies that maximize the effective delivery of great customer service. For example, management may ensure ample floor coverage by always having a staff member available to serve facility members and guests. In addition, you might also provide simple tangible amenities that set you apart, and above your competitors (*i.e.*, provide toiletries in locker rooms, hand out cooled workout towels and a bottle of water to members as they walk out onto the workout floor). For staff, they follow the "excellence in service" paradigm when performing their work activities. If a member asks where the workout towels are, the employee doesn't advise the member and point to the pile of towels. Instead, he actually walks over to the pile, picks one up, and hands it to the member, asking: "Is there anything else I can get you?"

Having well-thought-out business statements like these will make it easy for you to develop effective business policies, and will give your employees a paradigm from which to act and make decisions that will impact your everyday activities. Keep in mind that to pull this off you need to make sure everyone is on the same page. Staff training becomes paramount the more dependent you are on your mission statement or core values. Disclosure of business policies and a "Member's Bill of Rights" is important to make sure that your members and guests are aware of what to expect and what is expected. Maintaining an environment of "like minds," ensuring that members, employees, and management are all on the same page, will help provide for smooth business operations.

Professional Standards

In addition to a business's own mission, vision, and values, fitness professionals are also guided by professional standards and guidelines provided by their credentialing organization. The ACSM provides such standards for its credentialed fitness professionals. Box 7.1 lists the Code of Ethics for ACSM-certified and registered professionals. Following such standards ensures the safe and effective delivery of professional services, as well as minimizing a fitness professional's exposure to liability.

BOX 7.1	CODE OF ETHICS FOR ACSM-CERTIFIED AND REGISTERED PROFESSIONALS

Purpose

This Code of Ethics is intended to aid all certified and registered American College of Sports Medicine Credentialed Professionals (ACSMCPs) to establish and maintain a high level of ethical conduct, as defined by standards by which an ACSMCP may determine the appropriateness of his or her conduct. Any existing professional, licensure, or certification affiliations that ACSMCPs have with governmental, local, state, or national agencies or organizations will take precedence relative to any disciplinary matters that pertain to practice or professional conduct.

This Code applies to all ACSMCPs, regardless of ACSM membership status. Any cases in violation of this Code will be referred to the ACSM Committee on Certification and Registry Boards (CCRB).

Responsibility to the Public

- ACSMCPs shall be dedicated to providing competent and legally permissible services within the scope of the KSAs of their respective credential. These services shall be provided with integrity, competence, diligence, and compassion.
- ACSMCPs provide exercise information in a manner that is consistent with evidence-based science and medicine.

(Continued)

CODE OF ETHICS FOR ACSM-CERTIFIED AND REGISTERED PROFESSIONALS (*Continued*)

- ACSMCPs respect the rights of clients, colleagues, and health professionals, and shall safeguard client confidences within the boundaries of the law.
- Information relating to the ACSNCP-client relationship is confidential and may not be communicated to a third party not involved in that client's care without the prior written consent of the client or as required by law.
- ACSMCPs are truthful about their qualifications and the limitations of their expertise and provide services consistent with their competencies.

Responsibility to the Profession

- ACSMCP's maintain high professional standards. As such, an ACSMCP's should never represent himself or herself, either directly or indirectly, as anything other than an ACSMCP unless he or she holds other license/certification that allows him/her to do so.
- ACSMCPs practice within the scope of their KSAs. ACSMCPs will not provide services that are limited by state law to provision by another health care professional only.
- An ACSMCP must remain in good standing relative to governmental requirements as a condition of continued credentialing.
- ACSMCPs take credit, including authorship, only for work they have actually performed and give credit to the contributions of others as warranted.
- Consistent with the requirements of their certification or registration, ACSMCPs must complete approved, additional educational course work aimed at maintaining and advancing their KSAs.

Principles and Standards for Candidates of the Certification Exam

Candidates applying for an ACSM credentialing examination must comply with candidacy requirements and, to the best of their abilities, accurately complete the application process.

Public Disclosure of Affiliation

Any ACSMCP may disclose his or her affiliation with ACSM credentialing in any context, oral or documented, provided it is currently accurate. In doing so, no ACSMCP may imply college endorsement of whatever is associated in context with the disclosure, unless expressively authorized by the college. Disclosure of affiliation in connection with a commercial venture may be made provided the disclosure is made in a professionally dignified manner; is not false, misleading, or deceptive; and does not imply licensure or the attainment of specialty or diploma status. ACSMCPs may disclose their credential status. ACSMCPs may list their affiliation with ACSM credentialing on their business cards without prior authorization (ACSM certified Personal Trainer[SM] [CPT], ACSM Certified Group Exercise Instructor[SM] [GEI], ACSM Certified Health Fitness Specialist[SM] [HFS], ACSM Certified Clinical Exercise Specialist®

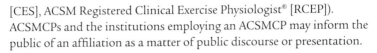

[CES], ACSM Registered Clinical Exercise Physiologist® [RCEP]). ACSMCPs and the institutions employing an ACSMCP may inform the public of an affiliation as a matter of public discourse or presentation.

Discipline

Any ACSMCP may be disciplined or lose his or her certification or registry for conduct which, in the opinion of the Executive Committee of the ACSM CCRB, goes against the principles set forth in this code. Such cases will be reviewed by the ACSM code. Such cases will be reviewed by the ACSM Committee on Ethics and Professional Conduct, which will include a liaison from the ACSM CCRB as appointed by the Chair of the CCRB. The ACSM CCRB will make an action recommendation to the Executive Committee of the ACSM CCRB for final review and approval (1).

Potential Areas of Professional Liability

Legal considerations impact many aspects of a fitness professional's experience. Areas of potential exposure for liability include the physical setting where program activities occur; the equipment used; the nature and quality of training techniques, advice, and services rendered; the degree of emergency preparedness and responsiveness; and the method of keeping and protecting records. While legal principles affect the training environment, as a practical matter, most cases today are settled out of court and therefore never actually create case law. To help fitness professionals to understand the practical ramifications, the following sections include the most common types of incidents likely to occur during day-to-day business. The application of legal concepts such as negligence to particular circumstances is then examined and the role of professional standards, guidelines, position statements, and recommendations from professional organizations is considered.

Safe Premises

While most fitness professionals focus on educating themselves on the latest training techniques and aspects of program design, in reality, fitness professionals are most vulnerable to professional liability for incidents that result from conditions of the physical setting where program activities occur. In general (2), any business owner who allows people to enter upon a land or into a building is required to provide a reasonably safe environment under theories of tort law. The area of tort law that regulates these issues is termed premises liability. The ACSM (3) has identified six fundamental standards to which facilities must adhere (see Box 7.2). Since a fitness professional may offer services in a variety of locations including a health and fitness facility, the outdoors, or in a client's home, the fitness professional should take basic precautions to ensure that every training setting is safe. (See "Your Resources" for suggested resource, ACSM's Health/Fitness Facility Standards and Guidelines, 3rd edition.)

Slip and Fall

The number one claim against fitness facilities and professionals is for injuries related to falls on the training premises, according to many insurance providers. Courts have consistently held that clients are entitled to "safe" conditions. Fitness professionals can foster safe conditions by a regular practice of inspection for, and correction and warning of any hazards in the workout and access areas to the workout location (5). For example, if items are on the floor that may cause a fall, the fitness professional should clear these away before beginning the session. If a group exercise class transitions into a classroom immediately following another class where participants' sweat collects on floor surfaces, the group exercise instructor must make sure that the floor is wiped dry before beginning the class. If safety conditions require, it is always better to be conservative and reschedule rather than to continue training in the presence of known dangers. Fitness instructors who work in aquatics facilities need to be particularly vigilant about deck conditions and pool access areas, since wet surfaces increase the likelihood of a slip-and-fall incident.

In addition to routinely inspecting locations before and during training sessions, fitness professionals should follow a procedure of proper equipment storage when equipment is not in use. Regardless of the exercise setting, encourage

---

| BOX 7.2 | **ACSM STANDARDS OF CARE FOR HEALTH AND FITNESS FACILITIES (4)** |

1. A facility must be able to respond in a timely manner to any reasonably foreseeable emergency event that threatens the health and safety of facility users. Toward this end, a facility must have an appropriate emergency plan that can be executed by qualified personnel in a timely manner.
2. A facility must offer each adult member a preactivity screening that is appropriate to the physical activities to be performed by the member.
3. Each person who has supervisory responsibility for a physical activity program or area at a facility must have demonstrable professional competence in that physical activity program or area.
4. A facility must post appropriate signage alerting users' to the risks involved in their use of those areas of a facility that present potential increased risk(s).
5. A facility that offers youth services or programs must provide appropriate supervision.
6. A facility must conform to all relevant laws, regulations, and published standards.

designating specific storage places for equipment so items are not left where people can trip over them. Different types of equipment require different types of storage. Make sure to use storage practices that not only store equipment effectively out of people's way, but also protect it from being used for inappropriate purposes. For example, many types of personal training equipment are attractive to young children and may be best stored in locked cabinets if children potentially have access.

Fitness professionals should also educate clients about appropriate clothing and footwear to prevent injury and to enhance training. Clothing should be comfortable, breathable, and allow for movement. In particular, fitness professionals need to check footwear and not allow clients to train with inadequate shoes. Factors such as poor fit, excess wear, and unsuitability to the activity all increase the risk of injury. An awareness of foot care issues is also important if the fitness professional works with clients who have certain conditions like diabetes. If the fitness professional works with people who are new to exercise, he or she may want to create a client handout that outlines appropriate exercise apparel and other exercise safety issues. If the fitness professional trains clients in a setting where protection is necessary, such as a helmet for cycling or pads for inline skating, the fitness professional should make sure that the client wears protective equipment (5).

Equipment Use

According to insurance providers, the second leading reason for claims against fitness professionals is injury resulting from use of equipment (5). These cases are based on legal theories from tort law that a fitness professional's duty or standard of care is to exercise reasonable care that the client does not suffer injury. If a fitness professional fails to take reasonable precautions, which is determined based on an evaluation of facts surrounding an incident, the fitness professional could be deemed to be negligent and therefore liable or responsible. Professional organizations such as the ACSM and National Strength and Conditioning Association also offer industry guidelines relating to matters of facility and equipment setup, inspection, maintenance, repair, and signage. While these standards and guidelines do not have the force of law, they can be introduced as evidence of the fitness professional's duty or standard of care. Keep in mind that the law does not envision that accidents never happen; laws exist to encourage proactive safe behavior to avoid preventable accidents.

As a practical matter, when it comes to using equipment safely, the question then becomes: What steps can fitness professionals take to prevent foreseeable accidents? Fitness professionals should always use safe, reliable, and appropriate equipment and use equipment for its intended purposes according to manufacturer guidelines (5). Members should only use equipment that is owned by the business or fitness facility. If a fitness instructor brings in his or her own personal equipment for use with a client, it may present additional liability. Whenever a fitness professional directs a client to use equipment, the fitness professional should provide proper instructions and supervision. In addition, policies and procedures for routine safety inspections, maintenance, and repair should be in place and observed systematically. Fitness professionals or facility managers should keep written records to demonstrate compliance with these policies and procedures. All of these steps are likely to minimize the risk of an accident. And, if an accident occurs and everything has been done to prevent it, then it is likely to be considered the type of accident that could not have been prevented by taking reasonable precautions.

Many clients will ask fitness professionals to recommend equipment. It is important for the fitness professional to work only with reliable fitness equipment dealers when recommending equipment to clients. If the fitness professional does not have a reliable vendor with whom to work, he or she should not recommend one piece of equipment over another. The topic of product liability is complex and outside the scope of this chapter. However, the fitness professional should be warned that equipment product managers are now pursuing clubs and fitness professionals for improper installation and maintenance in cases where they lose under product liability (5).

Free Weights

For a concrete example of potential liability for client injury from equipment use, consider this common scenario that involves an experienced fitness professional supervising an apparently healthy client who is performing a squat or similar exercise with free weights. The fitness professional encourages the client to use a heavier weight and to perform more repetitions even though the client complains of fatigue. The client suffers a debilitating back injury and sues the fitness professional and fitness facility.

Under theories of negligence, the fitness professional owes this client a duty to exercise reasonable care to prevent injury. Reasonable steps that a fitness professional can take to avoid this type of incident include fostering open communications with the client to encourage feedback and listening when the client communicates that he or she is reaching fatigue. Fitness professionals should know how to spot signs of fatigue and be conservative when implementing program progressions.

Another step that a fitness professional could take is to keep detailed records of numbers of repetitions, sets, and weight loads on specific training days. In this manner, a client can follow a reasonable plan of progression that minimizes injury risk. Before implementing progression in a program, fitness professionals can discuss the client's feeling of readiness to increase intensity and further evaluate whether the timing is appropriate for such a change. If specific records are maintained, the fitness professional is also in a position to evaluate whether or not a client's response to a particular exercise session is abnormal and requires referral to a physician (5).

Weight Machines

Even though machines carry a reduced risk of injury because the client's body is more stable and movement is more restricted than with free weights, injuries still occur. Most injuries happen when a client is encouraged to handle a weight that is too heavy; a weight plate slips and falls because a pin was not properly inserted; or a cable breaks. Weight plates have fallen and crushed ankles and feet, or hit people in the head. Clients suffer physical injuries and sue the fitness professional, fitness facility, and equipment manufacturer.

Here again, a fitness professional can exercise reasonable care to ensure that the client does not suffer this type of injury through a consistent practice of regular inspections and correction of any known hazards such as worn or faultily maintained equipment and through record-keeping of what weight the client has been able to lift, the number of repetitions, and sets and through following a conservative plan to increase intensity in close communication with the client. When working with weight training equipment, the fitness professional can develop a procedure of instruction and supervision for each exercise that includes an equipment and body scan to check for proper equipment setup and body alignment. Creating this type of instructional technique so that an inspection becomes a routine part of each and every exercise can go a long way toward preventing accidents.

Factors that courts have looked at in equipment-related cases include whether or not the equipment has been maintained appropriately and used for its intended purpose per specific manufacturer specifications. In particular, courts examined whether or not parts had been replaced in a timely manner and whether or not facility owners had insured that routine inspections and maintenance were conducted and documented (5). Regardless of the setting, a fitness professional should be proactive in learning about equipment safety inspections, maintenance, and record-keeping policies as well as the procedures for reporting the need for repairs. Before putting a client on any piece of equipment, the fitness professional should have first-hand knowledge of its readiness for use.

Keep in mind that courts also examine appropriateness of use. In one case, hotel management had placed equipment in a hotel gym that was intended for private home use. The court found the hotel liable for injuries suffered by the client. A training facility should provide commercial equipment; manufacturers do not design home equipment to withstand the wear and tear of frequent use by multiple users. If a fitness professional owns or manages a training studio, he or she should use professional equipment. Some manufacturers do produce "light commercial" equipment for facilities that are not heavily utilized like personal training studios and small, unsupervised hotel fitness rooms. However, it remains prudent to err on the conservative side and opt on commercial equipment in these unique settings. It is also important to be aware of any equipment class requirements that the facility's liability insurance policy demands. Any such gray areas need to be clarified prior to launching business operations.

Cardiovascular Machines

Treadmills are currently among the most popular form of exercise equipment in fitness facilities. Numerous cases feature instances where a client loses control and falls from a treadmill. These cases often involve middle-aged or older adult clients who are unfamiliar with the machine's workings and unable to keep up with the movement speed. Consequences from falls include back, neck, shoulder, and other joint injuries, broken bones, and even death. Clients (or their survivors) sue the fitness professional, fitness facility, and equipment manufacturer (5).

Of course these examples should not discourage a fitness professional from using equipment to condition clients. Equipment is an essential part of creating effective training programs. These incidents simply underscore the fact that whenever equipment is being used, fitness professionals must remain alert to the special risks presented and take proactive steps to manage and minimize these risks. And, fitness professionals should maintain detailed records to document the steps that have been taken. A detailed record of a given piece of equipment from date of installation with detailed maintenance service dates and documentation, along with any specific staff training documentation on proper use, and noted observations of wear or malfunction, etc. are examples of prudent documentation measures that minimize risk.

Scope of Practice

Another important area of potential liability for the fitness professional pertains to scope of practice. As fitness professionals work more closely together with health care providers to deliver a continuum of care to individuals, it is important to define respective roles. According to the ACSM's Code of Ethics for certified and registered professionals: "[Fitness professionals] practice within the scope of their knowledge, skills, and abilities. [Fitness professionals] will not provide services that are limited by state law to provision by another health care professional only"(1). This is particularly true of fitness professionals with advanced academic degrees or training and when working with clients who may have special exercise considerations. Both criminal and civil actions are possible for practicing without a license. Injunctions against a fitness professional's practice are possible. An elevated standard of care is required because malpractice is certainly a viable concern.

The contemporary delivery of health care services itself is in a state of flux due to high costs and attempts to reduce costs by expanding the roles of paraprofessionals in the medical context. As a result, states vary widely on what constitutes the practice of medicine and what is appropriate behavior for a nurse, physician assistant, or other paraprofessional. According to fitness law experts David L. and William G. Herbert, many states have defined the practice of medicine broadly so that persons engaged in exercise testing and prescription activities could, under some circumstances, fall within the range of such statutes (6).

Fitness professionals, therefore, need to become familiar with the relevant guidelines for scope of practice that are established at their affiliated organizations and institutions. For fitness professionals who operate their own businesses, it would be wise to seek the advice of local counsel and to take all other steps to manage risk effectively such as maintaining certifications, obtaining releases and waivers or consents as applicable, carrying liability insurance, clearly following accepted standards of care, and keeping detailed written records.

Supplements

Claims related to violations of scope of practice occur frequently in the area of nutritional supplements. A high-profile case brought against a fitness professional and a large fitness chain involved a scenario in which a fitness professional sold supplements, including one that contained ephedra, to a client. The client, who had hypertension, died. Survivors filed a suit. In another example, a fitness professional sold steroids to a client, who later suffered adverse consequences and filed a claim against the fitness professional (5).

In another incident, a personal training company combined supplement sales with its fitness packages to increase revenue. The company eventually had a client who was allergic to an ingredient in the supplement. The problem was compounded when the client assumed that if she took more than the recommended dosage, she would see more results. She ended up in the hospital, and even though she had been a loyal client for some time, she sued the fitness professional and the business. The case was settled out of court and the fitness professional lost his business. The problem was not that the fitness professional had sold the client the products, but that he had given her a written plan specifying what to eat and when to take the supplements. The fact that the client overdid it did not matter (5).

According to insurers, the problem with supplements is worsened by the fact that most supplement manufacturers do not carry any insurance coverage. Therefore, the people selling the supplements do not have any products liability coverage. Furthermore, most of the insurance policies for fitness professionals do not include protection for products liability.

In today's market, no one, even professional registered dietitians, can be certain about the ingredients in many supplements because they are not subject to government regulation. In addition, one can never be certain regarding who may have severe allergic reactions, including the risk of death, to any particular ingredient. To proactively protect client safety and to minimize the risk of professional liability, fitness professionals should avoid selling supplements.

Medical or Dietary Advice

No cases have yet been litigated to conclusion that involved a client suing a fitness professional for faulty medical or dietary advice, except in the case of supplements. However, remember that health care is a highly regulated area. The consequences of stepping over the line into the protected area of a licensed health care practitioner — such as a medical doctor, physical therapist, registered dietitian, or chiropractor — vary by state. You are exposed to potential liability for acting outside the scope of practice if your "advice" could be interpreted as the unauthorized practice of medicine and if this advice results in a client injury. The fitness professional should develop a comprehensive network of allied professionals and actively refer clients who request or require specialized services to the appropriate health care provider (5).

Fitness professionals should also learn to convey health-related concerns appropriately. For example, if a client's blood pressure measures on the high side during an evaluation, avoid saying "You have high blood pressure." Instead, suggest "your blood pressure is measuring a bit high today." If a client has an apparent injury, instead of saying "You sprained your ankle," say "from my experience you may have sprained your ankle." Fitness professionals do not diagnose medical conditions. Communicating accordingly with a client will help keep the fitness professional within their scope of practice.

Sexual Harassment

Sexual harassment claims represent another area of potential exposure to liability that is seeing growth in the number of claims against fitness professionals according to insurance providers. Since the personal training relationship can seem "intimate," it lends itself to creating more opportunity for abusive conduct on the part of the fitness professional or for a misinterpretation of actions on the part of the client. Numerous cases involve a male fitness professional and a female client. The female client believes inappropriate touching has occurred and that she has been violated. Or a personal relationship develops between the fitness professional and the client that then raises questions about the legitimacy of the business services rendered. The client believes undue influence was used to create an exploitive situation.

Sexual harassment is difficult to prove and often rests on credibility. Fitness professionals, therefore, should be vigilant to act professionally at all times. One strategy to protect against a claim of inappropriate touching is to always ask a client for permission to use tactile spotting, and to avoid it unless absolutely necessary. Some fitness professionals do not touch clients directly, but spot them through the use of another prop, such as a ball. Also, avoid situations behind closed doors where no one else is present. For example, if skinfold body composition assessments are offered, conduct the procedure in a room with other fitness professionals, perhaps behind a folding screen, or have another fitness professional or staff member present. If a personal relationship develops with a client, discontinue the professional relationship and refer the client to another fitness professional (5) (see Box 7.1 ACSM Code of Ethics).

Proper Qualifications

While no specific case on the books holds that fitness professionals have a higher standard of care based on their specific training in individual assessment, program design, and supervision, clients file claims after injuring themselves, based on the fact that a personal trainer does not have the qualifications represented in a facility's advertising literature. This claim is based on a theory of breach of contract since the facility failed to provide fitness professionals with the level of qualification that it has promised (5).

The best evidence that a fitness professional can show that his or her training services meets professional standards is to maintain certification and to conduct business according to the knowledge, skills, and abilities (KSAs) that are expected as minimum competencies by the certifying organization. For example, the ACSM-certified personal trainer[SM] (CPT) is defined as a fitness professional involved in developing and implementing an individualized approach to exercise leadership in healthy populations and/or those individuals with medical clearance to exercise. This certified professional is deemed to be proficient in writing appropriate exercise recommendations, leading and demonstrating safe and effective methods of exercise, and motivating individuals to begin and to continue their healthy behaviors.

The issue of a fitness professional's responsibility for advising appropriate levels of training intensity is even more critical as more people with special needs seek to work with fitness professionals. Fitness professionals who advertise their services to targeted clientele such as older adults or people with arthritis, claiming that they are trained to serve these niche markets, need to be sure that they are sufficiently prepared to serve these clients' needs. Evidence of sufficient preparation would include additional training and experience in working with people with particular needs. Fitness professionals should therefore keep written records of all certifications, continuing education, and work-related experience.

An important precaution to ensure that a fitness professional delivers services that are appropriate to the client is the prescreening health and medical history. In addition, the fitness professional needs to be able to assess risk and determine when a medical clearance is necessary. After all these precautionary steps are taken, the fitness professional needs to be able to conduct a safe fitness evaluation to determine the recommended level of training that will be safe and effective to meet the particular client's needs and goals. All of these measures should be kept in written records to document the steps taken by the fitness professional to create a specific exercise program.

The risk of exposure to liability for a fitness professional may be even greater when training services are delivered in a medical setting. In a 2003 Indiana case, a court held that even though a fitness professional was employed by a hospital and the fitness facility was owned by the hospital, the fitness professional was not a health care provider. The case, therefore, did not qualify as a medical malpractice case. The significance of this case, however, is that the client did try to sue both the fitness club and the hospital on the basis of injuries sustained while engaged in the personal training program, and the court did examine the fact that the training occurred in a setting with a close connection to a hospital. Another court might have found that this type of training did need to meet the standards of health care practitioners (5).

Emergency Response

As yet no specific case has involved a claim against a fitness professional for wrongful death in a situation in which a client has had a heart attack or other medical emergency and died while under the supervision of a fitness professional. However, since most fitness professional certifications require that fitness professionals have cardiopulmonary resuscitation (CPR) training (and some require first aid training and automated external defibrillator (AED) training), it is possible that a claim could be filed against a fitness professional who failed to provide an emergency response if that failure led to a death that could have otherwise been avoided.

ACSM and the American Heart Association (AHA) published a joint position stand in 1998 with recommendations for health/fitness facilities regarding the screening of clients for the presence of cardiovascular disease, appropriate staffing, emergency policies, equipment, and procedures relative to the client base of a given facility. In 2002, the ACSM and the AHA published a joint position stand to supplement the 1998 recommendations regarding the purchase and use of AEDs in health/fitness facilities (5). These organizations agree that a comprehensive written emergency plan is essential to promote safe and effective physical activity.

The AHA, the ACSM, and the International Health, Racquet and Sportsclub Association recommend that all fitness facilities have written emergency policies and procedures including the use of automated defibrillators that are reviewed and practiced regularly. Staff that have responsibility for working directly with program participants and provide instruction and leadership in specific modes of exercise must be trained in CPR. These staff should know and practice regularly the facility's emergency plan and be able to readily handle emergencies. In addition, these organizations encourage health and fitness facilities to use AEDs (5).

As evidence of professional competency, fitness professionals should keep CPR, first aid, and AED certifications current. A fitness professional should proactively familiarize himself or herself with any affiliated organization's emergency plan and be ready to implement the plan's procedures in case of emergency. For fitness professionals who operate a business, creating an emergency plan should be a top priority. Fitness professionals who provide training services outdoors or in a client's home should also have written emergency policies and procedures.

In addition to having an emergency plan, fitness professionals should also document any accident or incident immediately using an Incident Report Form (see Fig. 7-1). The fitness professional should include only the facts surrounding the incident and not any opinions regarding what may or may not have caused the incident. In addition, the names and contact information of witnesses should be included. And, the person who experienced the incident should sign the form, if applicable. Insurers will provide incident reporting forms and the fitness professional should always carry one to every training session.

Client Confidentiality

The failure to protect client confidentiality is another emerging area of potential liability for a fitness professional. This is rooted in the concept of preventing potential harm to a client's reputation. The fitness professional must keep detailed written records from the first client prescreening to notes documenting each training session. These records are critical evidence that can document that the fitness professional exercised reasonable care in performing his or her professional duties. At the same time, the fitness professional must exercise care to protect this information. The ACSM's guidelines for the fitness-testing, health promotion, and wellness area state that, "A facility should ensure that its fitness-testing, health promotion, and wellness are a system that provides for and protects the complete confidentiality of all user records and meetings. User records should be released only with an individual's signed authorization." Before a fitness professional discloses any personal information, even for marketing purposes such as a client testimonial, or "before and after" photos, the fitness professional should get and store a signed release form. Recently, a law passed by the U.S. Congress requires health care professionals to have strict policies regarding the safety and security of private records (the Health Insurance Portability and Accountability Act [HIPAA] of 1996, Public Law 104-191, which amends the Internal Revenue Service Code of 1986, also known as the Kennedy-Kassebaum Act). While it is still unclear if HIPAA extends to fitness professionals, it is wise to become familiar with this law and how it may impact the release of any personal information to a third party. In the very least, safeguarding a client's personal information is imperative to maintain one's professional integrity and should be part of a fitness professional's ethical standards.

INCIDENT REPORT

TO BE COMPLETED BY INSTRUCTOR

Date: _____

Location/Address of Accident or Incident: _____

Name of Instructor Completing the Form: _____

Date of Accident or Incident: _____

Approximate Time of Accident or Incident: _____ : _____ am   pm

Name of Injured Person: _____ Age: _____ Sex: _____

Injured Person's Address _____

City: _____ State: _____ Zip Code: _____

Home Phone #: ( ) _____ Work Phone #: ( ) _____ Cell Phone #: ( ) _____

How long has this person been under your instruction: _____

Describe the accident/incident: _____

Describe possible injury (sprained ankle, etc.): _____

Describe type of equipment involved: _____

List any type of treatment performed by you or by a doctor (include doctor, hospital name): _____

Were there any witnesses to the incident: yes _____   no _____

If yes, please have each witness write a brief statement about what happened.

YOUR SIGNATURE: _____

Figure 7-1. Incident report. Adapted from Jeff Frick, Fitness and Wellness Insurance Agency, 380 Stevens Avenue, Suite 206, Solana Beach, CA 92075.

RISK MANAGEMENT STRATEGIES

Risk management is an initial and ongoing process to identify relevant risks associated with the delivery of a service. This occurs through the application of various techniques, to eliminate, reduce, or transfer those risks through the

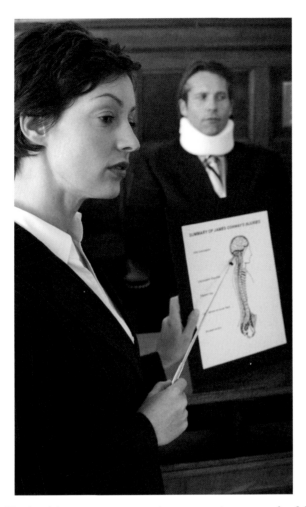

Figure 7-2. Effective risk management requires a proactive approach of thorough preparation and implementation of multiple strategies designed to minimize a business's exposure to liability. Reprinted with permission from American College of Sports Medicine. *ACSM's Resources for the Personal Trainer*. 3rd ed. Philadelphia (PA): Lippincott, Williams & Wilkins, 2010.

implementation of operational strategies to the program activities designed to benefit the clients and program (3).

Fitness professionals should manage risk exposure with a multilayered approach that incorporates five strategies. As the first line of defense, fitness professionals should create written policies, procedures, and forms that meet industry standards and guidelines and maintain detailed written records that document compliance with these policies. This strategy minimizes the likelihood that the fitness professional would fail to demonstrate that he or she exercised reasonable care under the circumstances. In other words, the fitness professional should make every effort to not be negligent (Fig. 7-2).

The second strategy involves using a release, waiver, or informed consent, depending on which legal document is recognized under the laws of the place where the fitness professional conducts business. A waiver provides for an assumption of risk. It is an acknowledgement by a participant, provided before beginning participation, to give up, relinquish, or waive the participant's rights to legal remedy (damages) in the event of injury, even when such injury arises as a result of provider negligence. Informed consent is a process that entails conveying information to a participant to achieve an understanding about the options to choose to participate in a procedure, test, service, or program. The purpose of these documents is either to demonstrate that the fitness professional fully informed the client of all of the potential risks and benefits of physical activity and the client decided to undertake the activity and waive the fitness professional's responsibility, or to demonstrate that the client knowingly waived his or her right to file a claim against the fitness professional even if the fitness professional is negligent. The fitness professional should keep these records indefinitely and in a safe place. Consent forms are not infinity contracts so provisions should also be made for an annual signing of these important documents. In fact, whatever documents are used in your preactivity screening process (*i.e.*, ParQ, Health History, Medical Clearance) should be "reused" on an annual basis, as participants' physical condition and health status change (3,5).

A third strategy is to carry professional liability insurance. This transfers the risk to the insurer. In that instance, even if the fitness professional is negligent, the insurance company assumes responsibility for resolving any claims. Most insurers of fitness professionals provide coverage for certified professionals. A fourth strategy is to incorporate the business to protect personal assets from any potential claims. A fifth strategy is to cultivate strong relationships with your clients and colleagues. Clients are much less likely to sue if they perceive a fitness professional as caring, responsible, and responsive to their needs. And, the final strategy is to consult local legal counsel to ensure that your business practices meet the requirements of your specific location.

Written Policies, Procedures, and Forms

The fitness professional should conduct his or her business according to written policies, procedures, and forms that ensure that his or her business practices conform to the standards set by professional organizations. In addition to developing a broad range of business policies, every fitness professional should also have risk management policies that include a written emergency plan and a preactivity screening procedure. The most important forms for a fitness professional include the following:

1. Member/Client Agreement (*i.e.*, Personal Training Contract)
2. Preactivity screening form such as a Physical Activity Readiness Questionnaire

3. Health History Questionnaire
4. Physician's Statement and Medical Clearance
5. Fitness Assessment or Evaluation Form
6. Client Progress Notes
7. Incident Reports

In the event that a fitness professional is encouraging a client to train independently on equipment in a particular fitness facility, an equipment orientation form for the client to sign to indicate that he or she has received instruction on the proper setup and use of weight training equipment would be useful to document equipment instruction.

Informed Consent, Release, or Waiver

In numerous states, courts are holding up waivers more and more as valid means of protection against litigation. In 2001, a California case was dismissed after a court held that the waiver form signed by a facility member when she joined protected the facility and its owners from liability when the member filed a lawsuit claiming that she slipped and injured herself. This case is consistent with other California cases (5). Depending on where a fitness professional lives, he or she may need to have a document entitled one of the following:

- Assumption of the risk
- Informed consent
- Release or waiver of liability

An assumption of the risk or informed consent document essentially explains the risks of participating in physical activity to a prospective client. The client then agrees that he or she knowingly understands these risks, appreciates these risks, and voluntarily assumes responsibility for taking those risks.

A waiver or release of liability document states that the client knowingly waives or releases the fitness professional from liability for any acts of negligence on the part of the fitness professional. In other words, the prospective client waives his or her right to sue the fitness professional, even if the fitness professional is negligent. A fitness professional needs to consult with an attorney in his or her location to determine which type of document is the standard practice for his or her state.

Professional Liability Insurance

In today's litigious environment, for the most protection, a fitness professional should carry professional liability insurance ($2 million per occurrence is the recommended amount), even when working in a business as an employee where the fitness professional may be covered under the business owner's policy. The reason for this is that it is not unusual for a single claim to result in a million dollar judgment. Purchasing the best protection enables the fitness professional to practice responsibly and feel confident that his or her business will not be destroyed by one mishap. (Most professional-certifying organizations recommend specific vendors. See "Your Resources" for two such randomly selected liability insurance vendors.)

Professional liability insurance provides a broad spectrum of protection from claims such as those arising from negligence, breach of contract, or even sexual harassment, and it can provide coverage for both injuries to a person or to property. Insurance professionals are expert at handling claims and will take care of all of the details, enabling the fitness professional to continue to operate his or her business (5) (see Box 7.3).

BOX 7.3   **KEY TERMS**

Contract law: Body of law that regulates the rights and obligations of parties who enter into a contract. A contract is an agreement between two or more parties that creates an obligation to do, or not to do, something that creates a legal relationship. If the agreement is broken, the parties have the right to pursue legal remedies. A contract can be written or verbal. The important elements of a contract include an offer and an acceptance, also referred to as a "meeting of the minds" and the exchange of something of value.

Duty of care: Refers to the level of responsibility that one has to protect another from harm. In general, the legal standard is reasonable care under the circumstances, which is based on an examination of factual details.

Informed consent: A process that entails conveying complete understanding to a client or patient about his or her option to choose to participate in a procedure, test, service, or program.

Negligence: A failure to conform one's conduct to a generally accepted standard or duty that results in harm.

Release or waiver: An agreement by a client before beginning participation, to give up, relinquish, or waive the participant's rights to a legal remedy (damages) in the event of injury, even when such injury arises as a result of the service provider's negligence.

Risk management: A process whereby a service or program is delivered in a manner that fully conforms to the most relevant standards of practice and that uses operational strategies to ensure day-to-day fulfillment, ensure optimum achievement of desired client outcomes, and minimize risk of harm to or dissatisfaction with clients.

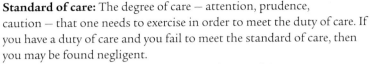

Standard of care: The degree of care — attention, prudence, caution — that one needs to exercise in order to meet the duty of care. If you have a duty of care and you fail to meet the standard of care, then you may be found negligent.

Tort law: A body of law that regulates civil wrongdoing.

From American College of Sports Medicine. *ACSM's Resources for the Personal Trainer.* 2nd ed. Baltimore, MD: Lippincott, Williams, & Wilkins, 2007, Box 22.1; p. 488.

CHAPTER SUMMARY

The fitness industry continues to grow and redefine itself as more health care providers acknowledge the need for exercise training as part of a program of preventive health care. Fitness professionals have great opportunities to work in a variety of settings and make a powerful difference in people's lives.

More professional opportunities, however, increase expectations of responsible professional conduct. More professional responsibility means more potential exposure to liability for failing to act responsibly. Today's fitness professional must understand these potential areas of risk exposure and the legal issues and industry standards and guidelines that surround these issues to deliver services confidently and to proactively manage risk. This professionalism in all aspects of doing business not only increases the personal and professional rewards of life as a fitness professional, but also ensures lasting business success amid the growing complexity of our modern legal environment. Ultimately, the purpose of liability is to protect individuals. The most successful fitness professionals will always keep in mind that rule #1 is to protect the best interests of the participant at all times and in all ways.

YOUR RESOURCES

Philadelphia Insurance Companies — Professional liability insurance vendor offering a variety of coverage options for fitness and wellness professionals including personal trainers, coach, dance instructor, martial arts, Pilates instructor, yoga instructors and life coaches, as well as fitness facilities.
http://www.phly.com/index.aspx
K&K Insurance — a recognized leading provider of sports, leisure, and entertainment insurance products. Provides coverage for a long list of fitness, sports, and recreation professionals, as well as equipment and facilities.
http://www.kandkinsurance.com

"Legal Aspects of Personal Training", ACSM Certified News: Bol 18: issue 2 2008. Tharrett SJ, McInnis KJ, and Peterson JA, editors. ACSM's Health/Fitness Facility Standards and Guidelines. 3rd ed., Human Kinetics, Champaighn (IL); 2007.

REFERENCES

1. American College of Sports Medicine. *ACSM Candidate Handbook, v7.0* [Internet]. Section F; 16-17. 2011 [cited 2011 August 21]. Available from: http://www.acsm.org/AM/Template.cfm?Section=Get_Certified&Template=/CM/ContentDisplay.cfm&ContentID=15683

2. Collins, JC, Porras, J. *Built to Last: Successful Habits of Visionary Companies.* New York: Harper Business, Division of Harper Collins Publishers; 1994.

3. American College of Sports Medicine. *ACSM's Resource Manual for Guidelines for Exercise Testing and Prescription.* 6th ed. Baltimore (MD): Lippincott, Williams, & Wilkins; 2009.

4. American College of Sports Medicine. *ACSM's Guidelines for Exercise Testing and Prescription.* 8th ed. Baltimore (MD): Lippincott, Williams, & Wilkins; 2009.

5. American College of Sports Medicine. *ACSM's Resources for the Personal Trainer.* 2nd ed. Baltimore (MD): Lippincott, Williams, & Wilkins; 2007.

6. Herbert DL, Herbert WG, Herbert TG. *Legal Aspects of Preventive, Rehabilitative and Recreational Exercise Programs.* 4th ed. Canton (OH): PRC Publishing, Inc.; 2002.

Going Solo

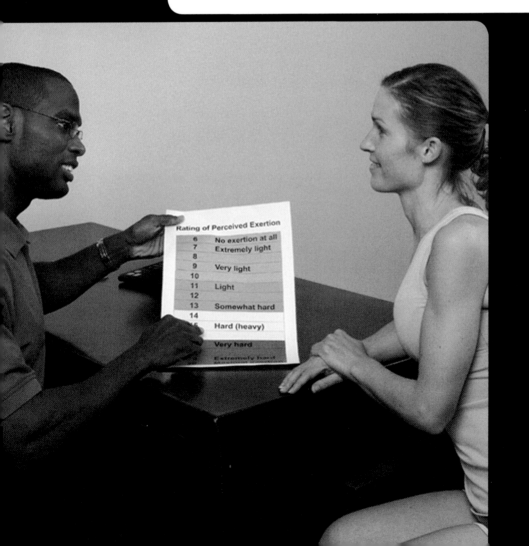

8

The Fitness Professional as Entrepreneur: Becoming a Business Owner

Chapter Objectives

After reading this chapter, the reader will:

- Understand a simple three-part question and answer process that will help the reader clarify his or her personal vision for his or her business
- Understand the basic business structures available to choose from
- Be able to select the most appropriate business structure to meet his or her individual needs
- Appreciate the importance of enlisting the help of legal and accounting professionals

GOING SOLO

After more than 30 years in the fitness industry, I can honestly say that I never met a personal trainer working in a fitness center setting who did not think "I can do it better." Many of those trainers have ventured off on their own only to, more often than not, come running back to employee status soon thereafter.

The fact is that being a highly skilled and knowledgeable personal trainer does not mean you will succeed in owning and managing your own personal training business. As seen in Part 2 of this book, the decisions made with regard to the type and size of a business, as well as its preferred structure, will require different levels of business-savvy and administrative oversight that can make or break any business and are not typically found in a fitness professional's repertoire.

STARTING YOUR OWN BUSINESS

The first step in starting your own fitness business is to define your personal vision for the business. Answering three simple questions can help put you on the right path.

- What is it that you want to provide in the marketplace?
  - What unique skills do you have that are marketable directly to the customer? Personal trainers, for example, can provide their training services, which may include fitness assessments, fitness program design, and individual or small-group training. Group exercise instructors may provide group exercise classes, which may include mainstream fare such as Step, Low-Impact Aerobics, or Sculpting classes, specialty classes such as Pilates Mat or Zumba, program-driven classes such as Silver Sneakers, or one-time-events such as "Master Classes." You might also think a little bigger and want to open a personal training studio, or launch a multifaceted, full-service health club.
- Where will you provide it?
  - Can you market your services to other business owners? For example, as a personal trainer, can you develop a symbiotic relationship with a local health club where you service their members, providing value for the health club owner, while the club provides you with a venue, equipment, and a membership base to market to? Do you want to provide in-home training where you travel to your clients to provide them your services? Will you bring small equipment to use with your in-home clients, or will you also provide your clients with a home-gym design service? Perhaps you want to start a boot camp program that you can deliver at a local park, or target corporate employees and negotiate the use of their company's corporate campus or parking lot where their offices are located.
- How will you provide it?
  - Will you serve under the health club's name or your own? Will you market your own services or can you negotiate some coop-advertising with the management of your "home facility"? Will you own and offer

your own branded monthly program of exercise classes at the local Community Center or Church basement, or perhaps partner with a local martial arts school, offering your training or group exercise programs during the morning hours, when the Dojo is closed or idle? Is your vision to build a fitness facility perhaps a large, full-service health club?

A personal trainer, for example, might want to provide his training services to a local health club as an independent contractor. This decision answers all three questions, providing for a simple business model that is likely to be a low-risk venture for the trainer. If, instead, the same personal trainer wants to open a small personal training studio, he will need to decide on location and size of business, which will dictate greater risk by way of an initial capital investment, and perhaps a more challenging business model. Launching a business of size, offering multiple services and requiring additional employees or workers can dramatically increase the risk to the owner and all stakeholders in the venture.

BOX 8.1   **THE U.S. SMALL BUSINESS ADMINISTRATION**

The U.S. Small Business Administration (SBA) (http://www.sba.gov/) was created in 1953 as an independent agency of the federal government to aid, counsel, assist, and protect the interests of small business concerns, to preserve free competitive enterprise and to maintain and strengthen the overall economy. The SBA helps Americans start, build, and grow businesses. Through an extensive network of field offices and partnerships with public and private organizations, SBA delivers its services to people throughout the United States, Puerto Rico, the U.S. Virgin Islands, and Guam. The SBA is also affiliated with the Service Corps of Retired Executives program. This program provides new business owners with an experienced mentor. This service is available throughout the country as part of the SBA.

Venturing out on your own presents different challenges to the fitness professional. As an employee, the personal trainer, for example, typically has professional liability insurance coverage by way of the facility's umbrella liability coverage. If the same trainer becomes an independent contractor at the same facility, servicing the same clients in the same manner, he must carry his own professional liability insurance, and oftentimes will be required to include the facility and or management as "additionally insured" entities on the trainer's policy certificate. Group exercise instructors are typically "hired guns" in a health club setting. Their job is to show up at a given time to teach a scheduled class, which can require different degrees of on-the-spot observational screening of class participants throughout the session. However, if a group exercise instructor decides to deliver a class independently, in the local Church basement or Community Center, the instructor should actually use some form of preactivity screening tool (*i.e.*, Physical Activity Readiness Questionnaire) to assess if it is appropriate for class registrants to participate in the class program prior to delivering any classes. In this scenario the fitness professional assumes the most risk, since they are responsible for all aspects of training and the physical environment may be out of their control.

CHOOSING YOUR BUSINESS STRUCTURE

Once you decide on your business offerings and model, you must select what business structure you will choose for establishing your business as an entity. There are a few basic business structures to choose from for a fitness business including, Sole Proprietorship, Independent Contractor, Partner, or Corporation (including Limited Liability Company, LLC).

Sole Proprietorship

In a sole proprietorship, one person owns the business. As the simplest, least expensive business model, often the only requirement before starting operations is a license or registration in the state and/or local city where the business will be located. Business profits carry over to the sole proprietor as personal income, and personal income tax is paid on any business earnings. Two drawbacks to this structure can be capital expenses for business start-up/expansion and personal liability for any incurred debt (1).

Independent Contractor

An independent contractor provides certain services for other individuals or businesses. Many personal trainers, for example, are independent contractors who provide personal training services to fitness facilities. This differs from the personal trainer who is an "employee" of the fitness facility. For example, the employee trainer's hours or work schedule are dictated by the fitness facility or business owner. The employee trainer gets paid via the company payroll having completed an Internal Revenue Service (IRS)-W4 form when hired, and receiving an IRS-W2 form after the end of the calendar year with an itemized breakdown of earnings and tax withholdings. The employee trainer provides services to the facility's members and clients as a staff member of the facility who manages the member's payments and is responsible for all accounting of those transactions. The client can pay the independent contractor trainer directly, and the trainer typically pays a percentage of his fee as "rent" to the club, or the client might pay the club for the services and the club pays the trainer his cut. Personal trainers who are independent contractors often work at multiple locations, set their own schedules, are paid by the session, and often have some control over training session format and fees. However, the percentage of the training fees that the individual contractor receives is negotiated ahead of time with health club management.

It is most wise for the health club management to file an IRS Form W-9 or Request for Taxpayer Identification Number and Certification. This form can be used to request the correct name and Taxpayer Identification Number (TIN), of the worker. A TIN may be either a Social Security Number, or an Employer Identification Number. The W-9 should be kept in the club management's files for 4 years for future reference in case of any questions from the worker or the IRS. Income tax filing should be done by the worker using the 1099-Misc — miscellaneous income form. All such income is taxed as personal income (2).

Partnership

A business partnership is formed by two or more people, either as an informal agreement or as a formal written document filed with the state government. It is recommended that all such agreements are reviewed by an attorney. This is the only way to ensure that the parties understand all aspects of the agreement and will be responsible in the event that the agreement dissolves. Partnerships are loosely governed by state and federal regulations and are subject to personal income tax based on each partner's ownership share. Forming a partnership allows for pooled financial resources and talents, but ownership transfer among partners may be difficult, and each partner can be held liable if the other partner fails to meet obligations.

Corporation

A corporation is a formal business entity subject to laws, regulations, and stockholders. Governed by a charter and bylaws, a corporation is a legal entity completely separate from its owners and managers. Investors, whose personal risk for financial liability is very limited, are often part of a corporation's start-up and growth. Corporation ownership can be more easily transferred than a sole proprietorship or partnership (1).

BOX 8.2

ONLINE INCORPORATION SERVICES

Online Incorporation Services – http://mycorporation.com – an online service owned and managed by business software giant, Intuit, provides access to its "Business in a Box," which includes everything from Articles of Incorporation to Simple Start edition of Quickbooks, to your Domain Name and logo design. Note that services like MyCorporation.com or Start-a-Business.com are mentioned here as available resources, but they are not endorsed in lieu of the advice of a legal or accounting professional.

Subchapter S Corporation

The subchapter S corporation, or S corporation, is a popular alternative for small businesses, combining the advantages of the sole proprietorship, partnership, and corporation. The benefits include

- Limited risk and exposure of personal assets
- No double taxation on both salary and business income
- Freedom for each partner to distribute dividends

S corporations are taxed as if they were partnerships – no tax is due on the entity level. Each partnership engaged in a trade or business must file a return on Form 1065 showing its income, deductions, and other required information. The return shows the names and addresses of each partner and each partner's distributive share of taxable income and deductions. This is an information return and must be signed by a general partner. The partnership does not pay any tax on its income but "passes through" its profits or losses to its partners. Partners must include partnership items such as their distributive share of income and deductions on their personal tax returns.

Limited Liability Company

An LLC is a business structure allowed by state statute. LLCs are popular because, similar to a corporation, owners have limited personal liability for the debts and actions of the LLC. Other features of LLCs are more like a partnership, providing management flexibility and the benefit of pass-through taxation. This means that owners report their share of profits or losses in the company on their individual tax returns. The IRS does not assess taxes on the company itself. This avoids the "double taxation" that general, or "C," corporations experience.

Owners of an LLC are called members. Since most states do not restrict ownership, members may include individuals, corporations, other LLCs, and foreign entities. There is no maximum number of members. Most states also permit "single-member" LLCs, those having only one owner. The federal government does not recognize an LLC as a classification for federal tax purposes. An LLC business entity must file as a corporation, partnership, or sole proprietorship tax return.

BOX 8.3   **HTTP://WWW.IRS.GOV**

http://www.irs.gov — a cornerstone web-based resource for any entrepreneur, this government Web site gives you access to every current tax form (and instructions for their use) you will ever need. It also provides a plethora of informational articles designed to help anyone starting a new business no matter how big or small your enterprise might be.

Always Hire a Professional!

Now that you have a clear vision of what you want your business to be, it is time to enlist the help of professionals. An attorney can help you file your business entity under one of the structures listed above. It is probably a good idea, however, to meet with an accountant first for two reasons. First, you will want to discuss the details of your business vision and your proposed business structure with the accountant, who will help you discern whether your thoughts are on-the-money. The business structure decision that you make can have some serious and far-reaching effects on your personal income taxes and overall finances, so you do want to run your business vision by him before making your final decision. The second reason for speaking with an accountant before you meet with an attorney is that regardless of your business structure and filing, you will need a federal tax ID number for your business entity. Note that it is a great advantage for a business to "connect" its accountant and attorney. Finding professionals who do or have worked together and specialize in working with small businesses is the best-case scenario. They are the professionals who can have the long-term vision most new business owners lack. They know what to look for in the long run and what to include in documents that will protect the business and its owner(s) in the future.

CHAPTER SUMMARY

Fitness professionals tend to be passionate about their practice and customers. It is this passion that makes so many of them want "to do it better." Developing your vision for your business can be a simple process of deciding what business services you want to provide the marketplace, where you want to provide those services, and how they will be delivered. Once you answer these three questions, you can likely decide under what kind of business entity you will operate, and launch developing more detailed business plans.

Enlisting the help of legal and accounting professionals is highly recommended, and using online incorporation or an out-of-the-box accounting program is no substitute for the guidance of an attorney or certified public accountant.

YOUR RESOURCES

Service Corps of Retired Executives (SCORE) is a Resource Partner with the U.S. Small Business Administration. It provides online workshops, business tools, and access to live mentors who offer free, helpful business advice online and through face-to-face mentoring at SCORE offices located throughout the United States.

http://www.score.org/index.html
http://www.irs.gov
http://mycorporation.com
http://www.Start-a-Business.com

The International Health, Racquet and Sportsclub Association (IHRSA) is the fitness industry's only global trade association. IHRSA represents over 9,000 for-profit health and fitness facilities and over 650 supplier companies in 75 countries. The value of joining such an organization cannot be overestimated. IHRSA Member Clubs enjoy full access to our information-rich Web site, publications and research, the industry's best meetings and webinars, member-generating programs, and the protection of IHRSA's government relations experts. *http://www.IHRSA.org*

REFERENCES

1. American College of Sports Medicine. *ACSM's Resources for the Personal Trainer.* 2nd ed. Baltimore (MD): Lippincott, Williams, & Wilkins, 2007.
2. IRS.gov. *Limited Liability Company (LLC)* [Internet]. 2010. Available from: http://www.irs.gov/businesses/small/article/0,id=98277,00.html

9 Developing Your Business Plan

Chapter Objectives

After reading this chapter, the reader will:

- Understand how to begin to more clearly define the reader's vision for the business
- Be able to identify the needs and processes necessary to launch the business
- Understand how to develop a basic capital expense, operating expense, and income budgets

SOLIDIFYING YOUR VISION

Once you have decided what your business is going to provide your customers, in what environment those services will be delivered, and what class of business entity you will be, you are ready to begin to solidify your vision and more clearly define your business.

Scope of Project

Where will you conduct business? Will it be within an existing business, or will you need to build-out a space and launch a stand-alone business? Will you be a one-man show or will you expand your reach through a staff of employees, other professionals who will deliver your business vision to your customers? Will you, instead, provide space for other professionals to utilize as independent contractors, and how will you negotiate a fee for your space? Will it be a straight monthly rent or a percentage of their revenue per session or service?

Large projects usually provide an advantage in economies of scale. For example, the larger your business space is, the lower the cost per square foot. Of course, construction, equipment, and operating costs will be dramatically higher. A larger facility means more space for more members. You may spend more on member amenities but your potential revenues in membership dues, for example, are likely to be higher if there is strong market demand. This is one of the many balancing acts you will have to do as a business owner/operator.

BOX 9.1   **PUT YOUR THOUGHTS DOWN ON PAPER**

The U.S. Small Business Administration provides an online tool called the Small Business Planner (http://www.sba.gov/smallbusinessplanner/index.html) that provides information and resources that will help you at any stage of the business lifecycle, from planning to launching and management, and even includes a free online course on how to write your business plan.

Location, Location, Location

Few things can ensure the success of a business more readily than being in the right place at the right time. Finding a location that provides an optimal footprint and space in which to deliver your services can be instrumental to your success. Making sure that this location is in an area where its demographics match well with your plan, and you are competitive with other like businesses can make the difference between boom and bust.

Demographics

It is important to conduct a thorough demographic study of the area in which you want to launch your business. Population, gender, age, and income are all related variables you must take into account before deciding that you are in the right area in which to launch your business. If, for example, you want to start a training program for adolescent athletes, and you are looking in a densely populated, affluent area that can afford your services, but households are mostly comprised of young couples between the ages of 25 and 35, it is not the best area in which to develop a program for adolescents, and thus might not be the right location to open your business.

The market range of your business, or "how far you can cast your net," is typically a 5-mile radius around your business. The more specialized your business services, the further your reach outside of your business location. For example, a mainstream adult fitness program will draw from within a 5–8-mile radius, while a specialized athletic training program for adolescents may draw from within a 15-mile radius. This is one reason why differentiating your business from your competition is important to your success.

BOX 9.2	**LOCATION, LOCATION, LOCATION!**

As you are "scoping the possibilities" of where you will launch your business, try identifying your top candidate cities by searching at http://factfinder.census.gov/. This U.S. government census Web site provides the most up-to-date demographic population data available, and can be searched by zip code. It will provide you with general information that you can use to weed out less desirable market areas on your list of possibilities. When you decide where you will launch your business, you will want to hire a local firm that can provide an in-depth demographic analysis of your target market, which you can then use in your final business plan to present to prospective investors in your business. (See the Demographics section of the Business Plan on page 180.)

Competitive Analysis

"Keep your friends close, but keep your enemies closer."
Sun Tzu, Chinese military strategist (1)

It is imperative that you have a thorough understanding of your marketplace before you launch your business. Identifying who your competitors are will help you better understand your customer, and analyzing their place in your market will help you set pricing, and develop programming and services. Keep in mind that there may be competitors in your area that provide services that differ from yours, but attract the same prospective clients. For example, you might be competing with a "Diet Center" for the same customers. You will also be competing with other entities that appear to provide similar services. These can range from other commercial fitness businesses to not-for-profit family fitness centers (*e.g.*, YMCA, JCC), to public community recreation centers. All of these organizations can vie for the same market that you are trying to attract to your business.

The simplest approach to acquiring information on your competitors is to shop your competition. It can be helpful to develop a "shopping list" prior to conducting the shopping to ensure you are focused on the right things. Visit the businesses of your competitors that are currently operating within a 10-mile radius of your desired location. Shop the business getting all of the information you can about their services, programs, rates, ancillary services, etc. Visit the competitor during a prime-time period so you get a sense of how busy they are during their busier hours. Be sure to tour the locker rooms and observe member amenities provided, number of showers and lockers, and assess things like cleanliness and the overall "feel" you get in the facility. Assess accessibility of the competitor. Are they on a busy road that is hard to access, is there enough parking for the demand, does it feel safe at night? How many trainers are out working the fitness floor, and how many are actually training clients? What is the business' menu of services that could offer additional value for the clientele for which you are competing? Get a schedule of their offerings — group ex classes etc. — to see their capacity.

After repeating this exercise at all of your competitors, you will be ready to compile all of the pertinent information. If you are planning a membership-based facility with personal training as a primary ancillary service, be sure to map out and compare everything from membership freeze and personal training appointment cancellation policies to program terms, rates, and services. Try to get a handle on trainers' qualifications, the membership fitness service model, and what members are expected to pay for above and beyond what's covered with their membership. Thorough price and service comparisons will help you develop your own menu of services, program rates, and policies and will help you develop programming providing "unique sales propositions"   a point of differentiation that will set you apart from your competitors.

Needs

Finding the perfect location sometimes means acquiring permission from the local government to launch your business in that location. For example, if you are looking for a large space, it would be to your advantage to find space at a modest cost per square foot. You would then bypass spaces that are designated for "office use" or even "retail" and look for spaces that might be designated as warehouse space, which come with a low cost per square footage and tend to be large spaces with high ceilings. The challenge, however, is that you will likely have to ask the town where the space is located to either rezone the warehouse space for "retail," or apply for a variance that will allow you to operate in the space as a fitness service business. Consideration should also be given to traffic flow near the space, public transportation options if applicable, or if the business is to be a destination parking capacity.

BOX 9.3   **DEPTH AND BREADTH OF YOUR BUSINESS**

- Before you decide on the size of your project, you need to develop an overall plan and scope of the types of services and programs you plan ·to offer. This will help you decide the staffing requirements, as well as facility and equipment needs.
- Develop a comprehensive initial list of all of the capital equipment you would ideally need to implement your intended programs and services, including costs. Capital equipment is an asset with an associated cost, have a life span of over a year (and will depreciate accordingly), and are typically required to perform or assist in producing a product, selling a product, or providing a service.
- Develop a staffing outline for your facility, including projected wages, salaries, and benefits; insurances; and staff levels and coverage needed.
- Develop initial specifications for your facility. Include different types of spaces and square footages of each. For example, the fitness floor and

locker room specs should be adequate to accommodate projected peak member and staff load, as well as the equipment you intend to purchase.

- Conduct a market analysis and competitive analysis to determine the optimal location for your facility. (See the Demographics and Competition Survey sections of the Business Plan starting on page 180.) Once a few optimal locations have been identified, begin looking for space in those locations.
- Compare lease rents, locations, and lease terms for the top three spaces. Use an attorney to help understand the lease terms of each landlord.
- It may benefit a first-time facility developer to research and hire an "owner's representative." This would enable the business owner to have an expert working on their behalf throughout the process.

Research an architect and possibly engineer (preferably professionals who have experience developing space similar to your business) while looking for suitable space so that when you find the right space, it is helpful to have the architect and engineers review the spaces as well prior to signing a lease to ensure feasibility.

- You can begin drawing up the tenant improvement plans with minimal delay.
- Once the best space is located, negotiate the best possible delay in making the first monthly rent payment and a landlord contribution for the tenant improvements. You should plan to complete construction and be open for business when you must make the first lease payment. Once you have discussed the lease in detail with your attorney, sign the lease and begin work with your architect on plans for construction.
- Make copies of the blueprints and apply for a construction permit with the city planning department. The permit process should include exterior signage as well, unless the landlord will provide it. Once the city approves the blueprints, begin soliciting bids from licensed and bonded general contractors.
- Select a contractor and begin construction. You should already have some ball park per-square-foot estimates as part of your start-up budget. You can now refine the architectural and construction costs estimate. Be sure to include some penalty clause for construction delays, or you will find that your project will invariably be delayed. Also be sure to add "contingency" capital to your start-up budget (typically 5% of start-up costs) in case there are overages.
- Apply for a business license with the city.
- Tightly supervise construction on a daily basis. This responsibility could be shared with an owner's rep.

Note that as soon as you can fill in the blanks of your capital/start-up budget, you should be securing the financing for your project. While the list above is in logical order as you progress through your business development and launch, you do not want to commit to a lease without having secured the start-up capital including operating costs to break even for your business.

Financials

Chapter 12 will delve deeply into how you can develop your financial plan, but before we get to that point in the business plan development, you should start thinking about your finances and how they relate to different parts of your business venture. The following outline will help develop your thought process prior to actually creating your budgets.

Establishing Your Capital/Start-Up, Operating Expense, and Income Budgets

Start-Up Capital   Once you have found a location for your business, you can begin to develop your capital expenses and start-up budget. It will include the cost of improvements (construction, fixtures, etc.). Gathering bids from general contractors will be helpful, as they will likely provide you with a cost per square foot that will cover all improvements. Professional fees may include an architect to develop drawings and a master plan for your space, and an engineer to figure out any pertinent issues like utilities, sewage/drainage, and a designer to design the exterior and/or exterior of the space (i.e., landscaping). It will also include all equipment, from office equipment and business software to fitness equipment and accessories.

In addition to the cost of improvements, space design, and equipment, your start-up budget will also include noncapital expenses such as payroll expenses to cover the cost of your employees prior to actual business operations, marketing expenses, employee uniforms, office supplies, rent security deposit, and member amenities (*i.e.*, towels, toiletries, etc.). It is also important to leave a line item space open for working capital. This extra start-up capital is devoted to covering expenses accumulated before you reach breakeven in your operating budget. You can estimate the amount required for working capital once you have completed your operating budget.

Operating Expenses budget

To establish an operating budget for your business, do the following:

PLANNING AHEAD

There is a sample Start-up Budget for ABC Fitness DBA Triad Fitness on page 186. Please note that when developing your start-up or capital budget, you will want to itemize each expense area in its own worksheet, which will feed into a Summary Page of your capital expense workbook. This will make it easy for a prospective investor to see where your start-up totals originate from.

Estimate business expenses (exclusive of employee compensation) needed to operate annually. Be sure and include these when creating your budget.

- Rent
- Debt service on investment capital/loans (if applicable)
- Transaction costs for monthly dues (EFT)
- Utilities
- Advertising/Marketing
- Gas/vehicle maintenance
- Taxes
- Liability insurance
- Telephone/T1/Cable (Internet)
- Uniforms
- Recruiting costs
- Professional memberships/certifications
- Conferences and training
- Business supplies (computer, office supplies, postage, printing, etc.)
- Fitness equipment and maintenance
- Client gifts/awards
- Legal and accounting fees

Income Budget

Developing realistic revenue projections is a simple exercise based on information that you gather from your market and potential customers, as well as your competition. Develop the framework for your business by listing out your primary income streams, decide pricing, and then project unit sales going forward. These projections will be instrumental once you've launched your business for sales goals setting and program management. Build this out on a month-by-month basis to ensure that seasonality is taken into account as well as including membership terminations on a monthly basis.

PLANNING AHEAD

There is a sample 5-Year Operating Budget for a small business, the Sports Training Center on page 197. Regardless of when your legal fiscal year begins and ends, it makes sense to develop your annual budget in a form that is easy to relate to for the reader. The included worksheets show projected income and expenses over a 12-month period and show year-end totals that carryover to the next budget page. This makes it easy for the reader to track income and expense figures progressively throughout your 5-year operating budget.

PRICING

Once the framework for the business is complete, specific pricing and budgets can be established. Typical direct expenses include salaries, payroll taxes, and benefits. Operational expenses include marketing expenses, program materials, and facility use charges. Pricing is typically established through consideration of a number of factors. It is essential to consider the general business objectives (*i.e.*, profit, overall client retention, projected number of clients, and average number of sessions per client per unit of time). To conduct programs within established budgetary guidelines, revenues and expenses should be reviewed regularly (2).

Ultimately, what a facility charges for membership or a trainer charges for training services is dependent on market forces. Completing a market analysis will help determine perceived value in the marketplace and thus, price point. Some key elements of a market analysis include

- Demographic study — How many potential clients are there in your geographical area?
- Competitive analysis — What are other trainers charging for their services?
- Consumer survey — What is your prospective client's perceived value? What do they expect to pay for your services?
- Demand projections — How large and dense is the market in your area?
- Financial considerations — Based on budgetary projections, what is the required revenue per unit sale? What volume is required to meet budget?
- Focus group information — What are the perceived needs of your prospect base?
- A market analysis will provide valuable information useful in developing an annual operating budget by supplying the baseline data to build the budget from the ground up. Personal training businesses typically begin with determining sales goals. The sales goals are set by determining the projected number of training sessions over the course of a week, month, and year multiplied by the average rate per session. These totals will help determine expenses over each period of time, since direct expenses correlate with sessions delivered multiplied by the cost per session.
- Budgets are necessary to forecast financial expectations and goals, provide accountability, track progress of actual versus projected results, and allow for justification and scrutiny. Completing an accurate, reliable, and analyzable budget without a computer is not easy. Simple software programs like Quickbooks or MYOB (Manage Your Own Business) are available and recommended, even for the solo trainer, that will help organize business finances and make their tax reporting easy (2).

- Although there are many resources available for the personal trainer/manager/club owner, it remains a prudent choice to enlist the guidance of legal and accounting professionals. The Internal Revenue Service Web site is a great resource for obtaining specific tax forms and information. It is accessible at: http://www.irs.gov/

CHAPTER SUMMARY

Once you decide the scope of your business, it is time to more clearly define your vision, and identify the needs and processes necessary to launch the business. Choose a location for your business based on demographics, competitive analyses, and market feasibility. Ultimately, that feasibility will be determined by your operating and income budgets, both of which will be market-driven.

YOUR RESOURCES

http://factfinder.census.gov/
http://www.sba.gov/smallbusinessplanner/index.html

Service Corps of Retired Executives (SCORE) is a resource partner with the U.S. Small Business Administration. It provides online workshops, business tools, and access to live mentors who offer free, helpful business advice online and through face-to-face mentoring at SCORE offices located throughout the United States.
http://www.score.org/index.html

REFERENCES

1. The Quotations Page [cited 2011 August 21]. Available at: http://www.quotationspage.com/quote/36994.html
2. American College of Sports Medicine. *ACSM's Resources for the Personal Trainer*. 2nd ed. Baltimore (MD): Lippincott, Williams, & Wilkins; 2007.

10 Structuring the Business Plan

Chapter Objectives

After reading this chapter, the reader will:

- Understand how to structure a basic business plan for the purposes of raising start-up capital, and manage and market his or her business
- Know some of the basic parts of a general business plan and what information to emphasize within each part

PUTTING YOUR VISION ON PAPER

There is nothing more important for any entrepreneur than laying out a clearly defined business plan. The plan serves the purpose of clarifying your vision and processes for your business, as well as putting your best foot forward to potential investors in your business. The ideal business plan has specific parts with clear objectives for both selling your dream and managing your business.

Cover Page

Like any business report or document, you want the reader's first impression to be a good one. You should always provide a cover page as the front cover of your business plan. Use the company logo, if you have already developed it, and add any pertinent tagline that further identifies your company, brand, or project.

Remember that your business plan is a valuable tool for your business and that it includes proprietary, confidential information. You will want to track each copy of your business plan. Do so by providing a space on the cover page of each copy of the business plan where you can number that copy, and keep a corresponding numbered log of each copy of your plan and for whom that copy was provided. Be sure to record the same copy number on the nondisclosure agreement signed by the recipient of the plan copy. Keep these and all business records and documents in a safe and secure place.

Legal Page

Immediately after the cover page, or even separate from the business plan document, provide the reader a nondisclosure document for him or her to sign and submit to you or the company, prior to reading the business plan. This nondisclosure document protects all of the information in your business plan as confidential and protected from further disclosure without expressed written permission from you or your company. Figure 10-1 below is a sample confidentiality and nondisclosure agreement.

Table of Contents

The next page should be your table of contents, where you clearly list the contents of your business plan in its entirety, which includes your marketing and financial plans. The following are some of the sections that might be included in a basic business plan.

The Executive Summary

The executive summary provides the most important points of your plan in an "at-a-glance" format. It should be brief and to the point, clearly defining the purpose of the plan, a description of the business, and should answer where the business will be conducted, who will be managing the business, and what unique features your business will offer. Also include a brief glance at the financial projections. Keep in mind that the executive summary is just that — a summary of the information detailed throughout your business plan. Keep it simple, clear, and concise, as this is sometimes the only portion that will be read by a potential investor. The executive summary has to provide enough information to "hook" and intrigue the reader to read-on and get to the details of your plan.

Business Objectives and Mission

These objectives should be specific and will help you set benchmarks for your business as you plan and reach milestones in your operation. Objectives may

---

Confidentiality and Non-disclosure Agreement

The undersigned reader acknowledges having received copy # _____ of ABC Fitness' Business Plan. The reader also acknowledges that the information provided by ABC Fitness in this business plan is confidential; therefore, reader agrees not to disclose it without the express written permission of ABC Fitness, Inc.

It is acknowledged by reader that information to be furnished in this business plan is in all respects confidential in nature, other than information which is in the public domain through other means and that any disclosure or use of same by reader, may cause serious harm or damage to ABC Fitness, Inc.

Upon request, this document is to be immediately returned to ABC Fitness, Inc.

Signature _____ Date _____

Name (typed or printed) _____ Date _____

This is a business plan. It does not imply an offering of securities.

Figure 10-1. Confidentiality/non-disclosure agreement.

include specific benchmarks that the business will achieve at specific milestone (*i.e.*, at the end of the first year of operation).

Your company mission should state and describe your general vision for the business. Use your mission statement to establish your business' fundamental goals for the quality of your business offering, customer satisfaction, employee welfare, compensation to owners, and so forth. A good mission statement can be a critical element in defining your business and communicating to employees, vendors, customers, and owners, partners, or shareholders.

For example, customer service experts frequently point out the need for a mission statement (see Chapter 7) that explicitly states the importance of customer service, so that employees understand how much the company values its customers. Quality assurance experts will also turn to a mission statement as a fundamental plank of quality control. A company needs to state its goals and priorities so the people charged with carrying them out can know and understand them (1).

Overview

The overview is where you detail the state of your industry and your company. Clearly outline your business objectives, including, when appropriate, a rationale for establishing your business in your desired space and location. The overview can serve, at times, as a needs assessment establishing your rationale for existing in your marketplace. This is also where you detail any specific unique products or services your business provides for your customers. Be sure to clearly outline target markets for any particular product or service.

Management

The next important portion of your plan includes a history of your management team. Be sure to describe what roles each will play and how specific past experiences relate directly to the success of your new business.

Departments and Concepts

This is a detailed description of the unique product lines and services your business will provide to your customers. Be sure to answer what the services are, detail how they will be delivered, what market niches are served by each individual service, and describe your vision for the marketing potential for each.

Staffing

Describe who your business will recruit for employment. Pay special attention to professional education and credentials for those employees that will provide professional services. Detail how you will recruit on board new employees, and how you will provide for their professional development throughout their tenure with your company.

Market Assessment and Competitive Analysis

This very important part of your business plan is where you identify the demographics of your marketplace, identify who your target market is, and detail who in the marketplace will challenge you for market share.

A demographic analysis is crucial to assessing if there are enough potential customers in your market area. Fact-finder at www.Census.gov is a great resource for age, gender, economic, and other general population data. Once you have a handle on the total number of potential customers within a 15-minute drive (typically 5- – 8-mile radius from your location), you want to complete a competitive analysis.

A competitive analysis will help you further define your customer, give you an idea of how to market to your customers, and how to price your services so that you are charging realistic, competitive rates and planning your budgets accordingly. Be sure to include rates, services, market niches, etc., for each of your product lines. Using the business plan shown later in this chapter, ABC Fitness has three distinct target markets. One of them, for example, is the adolescent athlete. You will want to include in this competitive analysis any after-school athletic training programs that target adolescents. These competitors might differ widely from those competitors in the adult fitness market — one of ABC's other target niches.

Marketing Plan

Here you want to further detail your market area using demographics data as well as anecdotal information collected from surveys, focus groups, and other information-gathering vehicles. Describe in detail how you will market your services, develop your brand, and, essentially, get customers in the door. List all of your projected marketing vehicles, describe any seasonal marketing approaches that you will use, and define who (if any) your advertising experts will be (*i.e.*, specific agencies, consultants, etc.)

Be sure to include your marketing strategies for both acquisition (acquiring new customers) and retention (keeping current customers) for each of your main product lines or services, and/or departments. Consider that it is typically more costly to find new customers than it is to keep your current customers, and once you "fail" your customer, and lose them as a result, you have lost them for good.

Use of Funds

This portion of your plan clearly outlines where start-up capital will be allocated in order to launch and continue to operate the business.

Financial Plan

The financial plan should include detailed capital and start-up budget, operational expenses budget, income projections, cash-flow and balance sheets for years 1 through 5.

Exhibits, Supporting Documents, and Data

Immediately following the financial data documentation, there should be a compilation of any other files that serve as supporting documentation. Any presentation files used in the selling of the business plan should also be included in hard-copy format in this section.

CHAPTER SUMMARY

Laying out a clearly defined business plan serves the purpose of clarifying your vision and processes for your business, as well as putting your best foot forward to potential investors in your business. The ideal business plan has specific parts with clear objectives for both selling your dream and managing your business. Your business plan tells prospective investors what your business is, who you are, and what your expectations for your business are. A simple, clearly laid out plan will help make investors most comfortable with your vision and plan for success.

YOUR RESOURCES

www.Census.gov
http://www.sba.gov/index.html
Business Plan Pro-a software application developed by Palo Alto Software (http://www.businessplanpro.com), will help take you step by step through the process of writing your business plan. It provides sample business plans in many different industries, and automated financial reporting.

REFERENCES

1. SBA.gov. Essential Elements of a Good Business Plan, 2011 [cited 2011 August 21] Available at: http://www.sba.gov/category/navigation-structure/starting-managing-business/starting-business/writing-business-plan/essential-elements-good-busines

Developing Your Marketing Plan

Chapter Objectives

After reading this chapter, the reader will:

- Understand how to collect and compile prospective customer data to utilize in the development of a comprehensive marketing plan

- Know the importance of combining different marketing vehicles in a collaborative, concerted effort to promote the business and any timely events or activities that will ultimately attract leads in through their front door

- Understand how to use a marketing calendar to plan and schedule all marketing events and vehicles from creative development, to submission, to publication

CREATING YOUR MARKETING PLAN

Your marketing plan defines and maps out the process that takes your marketplace information (demographics and competitive analyses), combines it with some direct prospective feedback (market survey, focus groups, community roundtables), and your business's vision and mission to develop and bring your products and services to the marketplace. The plan should be included as part of the business plan as well as summarized in its executive summary.

DEFINING YOUR BRAND

You should have a clear vision of who you are in the marketplace and who your customer is. If, for example, you sell luxury items like Rolls Royces, you need to locate your business where the household incomes of the surrounding population can afford to purchase your luxury items to support your business. Population density is one variable to factor in when deciding the location for such a business, but it must be coupled with economic status (household incomes) of that population. You need to have enough potential customers within your demographic to locate your business within that market area.

If, instead, you are a value-driven business with low-end price points, you need to locate in a densely populated area, knowing from the launch that your market share must support your overall business operations while considering the lower margins that you will contend with as a lower-priced value player. For example, if you are a XYZ Fitness charging $10 per month in membership dues, you might need 16,000 members to keep you afloat, while the Your Family Fitness facility 1 mile down the road targets 2,000 members at $80 per month. These clubs' revenues might be similar, but their target markets and unique selling propositions are dramatically different. Planet Fitness might appeal and market to the price-conscious consumer who does not feel the need for a lot of direction, and is simply looking for a "no-frills" place to go exercise. 24-Hour fitness offers programs and amenities, which may include group fitness classes, fitness assessments, and fitness program design. These services appeal to a different clientele, who might want a little hand-holding, or a more personal level of service. Personal training studio clients will expect a clean workout towel and a bottle of water at the start of each workout, along with the personal attention of their personal trainer throughout their visit. Canyon Ranch visitors expect an exercise studio floor that you can eat off and 600-thread Egyptian cotton sheets in their rooms if they happen to be staying for a few days.

The point is that regardless of your product and service offerings, you must have a target audience that your products and services speak to. Your marketing then is the language and modes by which you communicate with your market.

DEVELOPING YOUR PLAN OF ATTACK

Once you have defined your brand you will want to decide what methods you will use to "get the word out." A good place to start is to research and go through much of the local media looking for ads and promotions for products and services similar to yours. In some markets, local newspapers are standard effective advertising vehicles for fitness services. In other markets, newspaper advertising is a waste of money. Look for ads for fitness services that appear to closely match your brand and target market. This exercise is invaluable, because you will learn what your competition is advertising, as well as where. Chances are that if your competitor is always advertising in a specific local magazine or newspaper, they are getting some kind of return on that investment, and it might be worth a trial or "test" run.

TESTING YOUR MARKETING

No matter what advertising or marketing vehicles you use, you always want to measure their outcomes. Chapter 4 describes for you, in detail, many of the different marketing vehicles that are at your fingertips, and how to implement them. This chapter focuses on developing your plan of attack by piecing together some of these different vehicles to effectively market your products and services. Your plan should include different vehicles that vary in their reach and areas but target specific segments of your market. Once you implement your plan you should keep accurate statistics regarding the outcomes of all of your advertising and marketing vehicles. This can be as simple as providing a guest pass on the back of your business card and seeing how many you actually get back in prospect leads visiting your facility. It can also be assessing the return on investment of a newspaper ad. Tracking these numbers will help decide what to keep in the marketing plan for future investment, and what to drop out of this mix.

DEVELOPING YOUR MARKETING PILLARS

Regardless of what marketing vehicles are chosen, the business should be built upon multiple pillars or vehicles. Identify appropriate daily, weekly, and monthly media that fit the business brand and align with its target market. Decide on the support materials or activities that will have to dovetail or align with ads. For example, a monthly program based on National Heart Month (February) can be announced in a newspaper ad, free in-house lectures and heart-healthy recipes can be distributed to your e-mail list, and a guerilla marketing effort can include heart-shaped free trial passes, which can be distributed to commuters at the local rail station on their way to work. The idea is to have a concerted effort, with all vehicles aligned with the single purpose of getting leads in the door.

BOX 11.1	**OFF-THE-SHELF MARKETING PROGRAMS AND TOOLS**

There are currently several high-profile marketing tools companies specializing in the fitness industry. It is important to have a master plan developed before consulting with any such groups. Businesses will always have the opportunity to learn and be influenced in its array of marketing tools, but it doesn't necessarily want to "be sold" on something that was not part of its plan. Many of these companies are great at finding future clients (providing targeted mailing lists), and offer electronic and hard-copy off-the-shelf tools that can be used to market the business. Keep in mind that it might be a tool that the competition is already using, and if a business wants to differentiate itself from the competition, the last thing it wants to do is use marketing pieces or vehicles that "look the same" as those of its competitors.

Building the Business's Image

Business cards and professional letterhead are a must-have, whether you multipurpose them (*i.e.*, Free Guest Pass on the back of the business card) or not. Add a logo and a brochure to the business stationery and you have a powerful arsenal for building the business's image and brand. These standard items must speak of the brand and create a clear picture in the prospective customer's mind regarding what the business is and what its brand is about. Is it the Rolls Royce provider of fitness services, or more of a "Discount Fitness" type of facility?

Advertising

Whether you enlist the help of a professional advertising agency or create your own ads for your targeted media, you will want to include some basic timely advertising in your marketing plan. The ads can promote your standard products and services, or can promote specific time-oriented programs or promotions that you run periodically during specific times of the year. The primary goal of advertising is to reach "suspects" in your market, and make them prospects by developing them as leads. In other words, get them to inquire about your products and services. Once they inquire, it is up to you and/or your sales team to identify those who are qualified leads and convert them from prospect to customer. Keep in mind that advertising rarely "sells" your products and services.

Supporting Roles

Guest passes, gift or discount certificates, promotional flyers, guerilla market-ing vehicles and tactics, internal membership programs are all parts of your supporting pillars. Some may be used year-round, while others help drive interest to seasonal promotions. Special "free" in-house events can be the reason for prospects to come to your front door. Your advertising can promote your monthly or seasonal promotion, and a timely banner across the ad can promote a special event. Again, all of these are vehicles designed to develop your business's image or brand in your community, as well as provide you with viable leads.

THE MARKETING CALENDAR

Chapter 4 provides a sample 12-month marketing calendar that helps you, the business owner/manager, plan when different marketing activities should take place in order to launch timely and effective advertising campaigns and promotions. This is an effective tool to use when developing your marketing pillars. It will help you effectively space out your marketing efforts, making it easy for you to schedule and subsequently track the outcomes and returns on investments for each of your marketing activities.

Figure 11-1 shows a completed marketing calendar that includes the different marketing pillars, as well as monthly themes and promotions.

Note that this calendar can be further broken down so that you can schedule your creative and posting deadlines with different media. For example, if you plan on advertising in a newspaper on the 1st week in February, you can add a row to the calendar showing the creative or ad development phase, scheduling that for the 3rd week in January. Then add another row for the ad submission date on the 4th week of January. This process makes it easy for you to identify, schedule, and execute your marketing activities throughout the year.

CHAPTER SUMMARY

The marketing plan is the coordinated effort clearly defining how you promote your business to your marketplace. Demographic and competitive analyses data should be part of deciding where and how to market your business. Year-round "supporting materials" include guerilla marketing tools like business cards, guest passes, flyers, and discount/gift certificates. The marketing calendar makes it easy for the business owner/manager to plan and manage his or her concerted marketing efforts year-round.

Week	Jan 1	2	3	4	Feb 1	2	3	4	Mar 1	2	3	4	Apr 1	2	3	4	May 1	2	3	4	Jun 1	2	3	4	Jul 1	2	3	4	Aug 1	2	3	4	Sep 1	2	3	4	Oct 1	2	3	4	Nov 1	2	3	4	Dec 1	2	3	4
Events																																																
Save the Date																																																
Register																																																
Reminder																																																
Monthly Programs																																																
Resolution Solution																																																
National Heart Month																																																
Commit to Get Fit																																																
Bikini-Fit Challenge																																																
Get Healthy America																																																
Back-to-School																																																
Workout for Hope																																																
Customer Appreciation Holiday Party																																																
eNewsletter																																																
Facebook posts/ads																																																
Website Blog																																																
Newspaper Ads																																																
The Record																																																
The Suburban																																																
Magazine Ads																																																
201																																																
BC																																																

Figure 11-1. Master marketing schedule.

YOUR RESOURCES

Editor's Note: The inclusion of the following resources does not imply an endorsement of any kind. Each resource has a place in their market niche and can provide the fitness owner/operator with invaluable information and sales and management tools with which to operate their business. There are many such resources in the marketplace, and the inclusion of the resources below does not imply an endorsement over the use of another similar resource.

The Peak Performance International Fitness Network has been the leading provider of management and marketing information, as well as staff training and education, for the health club industry since 1984. They offer an array of marketing tools including Direct Mail campaigns, e-mail marketing, and mail to web strategies.
http://www.healthclubpros.com/

Bedros Keuilian is fast becoming a leader in the fitness marketing and sales education business, especially if your core business is personal training and/or fitness boot camp programs. His blog provides a broad collection of videos and case studies that will help any fitness entrepreneur in the development of their own marketing strategies.
http://ptpower.com/

The home of Net Profit Explosion (NPE) is the brainchild of Sean Greeley & Eric Ruth, who have developed an array of educational and management tools for fitness business operators.
http://www.fitnessmarketingsystems.com/

Private Label Fitness provides support materials for fitness and nutrition programs that can be private labeled with your own company logo and information. This can be part of your "retention tools" arsenal.
http://www.privatelabelfitness.com/

12 Developing Your Financial Plan

Chapter Objectives

After reading this chapter, the reader will:

- Understand some of the basics of writing a small business financial plan, including the importance of enlisting professional guidance from the business owner's accountant

- Know how to develop a simple start-up capital budget, an operating budget, and a P&L/income statement

SHOW ME THE MONEY! — WHAT EVERY INVESTOR WANTS TO SEE

Once a mission and vision are laid out step by step in the business plan, it is now time to begin developing start-up and operating budgets. These are crucial pieces of information that will add to the business plan when pitching banks for loans or investors for private equity. That said, make no mistake about it — that you should never prepare these documents without an accountant reviewing them prior to soliciting funds. In fact, it is most prudent to meet with an accountant several times throughout this process to make sure the financial documents are in order and, most importantly, clearly understood by you and anyone else who will be pitching investors on behalf of the business.

This chapter focuses, then, on two documents that are key elements of a financial plan. We briefly review the process by which a start-up capital budget and an operational budget can be developed. This later budget can also serve as an ongoing profit and loss (P&L) statement. It is highly recommended that cash flow (cash inflow and outflow over a period of time) and other financial statements are developed by a bookkeeping or accounting professional(s).

START-UP — CAPITAL AND NONCAPITAL BUDGET

A start-up budget is very simply a line-itemized listing of start-up capital and noncapital expenses. Capital expenses tend to be one-time expenses like construction or lease-hold improvements made on the business space, as well as large equipment that will last for at least 1 year, and are required to produce a product or deliver a service. Noncapital start-up expenses are "consumable" items like locker room amenities, staff uniforms, or office supplies. They will eventually fall into the base operating expenses budget, but it is obvious that launching the business will require an opening supply, so these items must be included in the start-up budget.

Construction expenses will typically be determined as a dollar per square foot estimate, which will be provided by the general contractor on any lease-hold improvements jobs. Large jobs may require the hiring of an architect and/or engineer. Allocate their fees and be sure to provide for a 5% swing in either direction (up or down) to serve as a contingency plan. The same goes for any professional fees directly involved with the launch of the business.

Future construction or lease hold improvements are "amortized" typically over a 10-year period. This is an accounting concept used to estimate the amount accrued over time necessary to pay for renovations or other lease-hold improvements. Capital equipment, on the other hand, is typically depreciated over a 7-year period, but can vary between 5 and 10 years. There are advantages and disadvantages to each, and the business accountant can set up the most advantageous budgetary factors to keep the business on track over the long term. Depreciation is an accounting and tax concept used to estimate the loss of value of assets over time. For example, treadmills depreciate with use. Depreciation serves as an income tax deduction that allows a taxpayer to recover the cost or other basis of a business asset or property. It is an annual allowance for the wear and tear, deterioration, or obsolescence of capital equipment property. Most types of tangible property (except, land), such as buildings, machinery, vehicles, furniture, and equipment are depreciable. Likewise, certain intangible property, such as patents, copyrights, and computer software is depreciable (1).

Figure 12-1 shows a start-up budget summary page for Triad Fitness, a large multipurpose fitness facility whose detailed Capital Start-up Budget can be found on page 186. It presents an idea of the items that need to be included in a large project of Triad's magnitude.

When developing this kind of financial document, it is recommended that available technology use be optimized. The simplest way to go about this is to use a spreadsheet program (*i.e.*, Microsoft Excel) and develop a workbook where single-page spreadsheets can be created that itemize every start-up expense, and whose totals get automatically added into the appropriate line item on the

	Total Square Feet		17,500				
	Construction Costs per Sq FT	$	75.00				
Capital Costs	**Budget**	**Total within each Area**					
Construction & Related Costs							
Construction Costs	$	1,312,500					
Construction Contingency: 5% of Cons't Costs	$	65,625					
Architects Fee: 10% of Cons't Costs	$	131,250					
Engineers Fee: 3% of Cons't Costs	$	39,375					
Signage — Internal & External	$	15,000					
Misc Consultants — Expediter, Graphics, etc.: 0.5% of Cons't Costs	$	6,563					
Sub-Total Construction & Related Costs			$	1,570,313		$	104,688
							10 Yrs Professional Fees
15 Yrs Amortization						$	10,000
							15 Yr
						$	114,688 Amortization
Exercise & Related Equipment	**Items to be Leased**						
Accessories	$	9,446					
Broadcast Vision	$	52,004					
Cardiovascular Equipment	$	227,559					
Computer & Office Hardware	$	35,739					
Computer Software	$	15,960					
Free Weights and Plate Loaded Equipment	$	35,216					
Group Classroom Equipment	$	28,187					
Laundry Room and Storage Equipment	$	19,372					
Selectorized Strength Equipment	$	108,828					
Athlete Training Center	$	25,477					
Testing Equipment	$	3,198					
Total Exercise & Related Equipment	$	560,985					
1st & Last Month Deposit on Lease			$	21,504			
							7 Yr
7 Yr Depreciation						$	80,141 Depreciation
Start Up Costs - Non Capital	**Budget**						
Locker Amenities and Hygienic Supplies	$	16,791					
Member Towels	$	13,488					
Staff Uniforms	$	2,200					
Office supplies	$	10,000					
Salaries							
Thorne — 6 months	$	37,500					
Milkin — 6 months	$	37,500					
Pirelli — 4 months	$	25,000					
2 F/T Ex Phys — 1 Month	$	6,251					
2 F/T Admin Assist for Adult & STA — 1 Month	$	4,840					
2 F/T LRA — 1 Month	$	3,987					
4 P/T Receptionists for Mon-Sun — 2 Weeks	$	1,328					
2 P/T LRA for Sat & Sun — 2 Weeks	$	440					
2 P/T Ex Phys for Sat & Sun — 2 Weeks	$	616					
Sub-Total Salaries			$	117,461			
Payroll Taxes 10%	$	11,746					
Advertising, Marketing & Promotion	$	45,000					
Professional Fees	$	50,000					
Rent Security Deposit	$	65,625					
Sub-Total Non Capital Start Up Costs			$	332,311			
Working Capital							
1st Year Requirements	$	200,000	$	200,000			
Total Capital Funds Needed			$	2,124,128			

Figure 12-1. Start-up budget summary page for triad fitness.

summary page. This way, it is easy for the owners or prospective investors to review the start-up budget and go back and forth to review each line item on its assigned page.

PLANNING AHEAD

Triad's complete start-up budget workbook is included in the Capital Start-up Budget section of the Business Plan on page 186. Note that ABC Fitness is doing business as (dba) Triad.

When developing a start-up budget, it is important to compile and calculate every expenditure that will be required to launch the business. The start-up budget should be completed after the initial operating budget, since any cash-flow shortfall in the project must be offset with start-up capital. For example, in Triad's case, there is an additional $200,000 added to the initial budget as operating capital that is included to cover cash-flow shortfalls until the new business is "in the black", and achieving positive cash flow.

OPERATING BUDGET/INCOME STATEMENT

When creating an operating budget, it is important that a "mental walk-through" of the facility be done in order to identify every possible operating expense and staffing need in order to come up with accurate estimates of expenses from day one. The operating budget will include all of the base operating expenses, the direct or staffing (payroll) expenses, and the revenue/income. It is also known as the income or P&L statement.

Figure 12-2 demonstrates year-1 of the operating budget/income statement for the Sports Training Academy; in contrast to Triad, this is a small start-up business that focuses on providing an array of fitness services including group fitness boot camps, personal training sessions, and a small group athletic conditioning program.

PLANNING AHEAD

The Sports Training Academy's complete 5-year budget and start-up budget can be found in the Five-Year Operating Budget section of the Business Plan on page 197. You will note the projected breakdown of revenue-producing activities outlined under each income total. These are based on realistic projections and depict the slow, but gradual growth of the business over the first 5 years of operations. Banks and/or investors typically will want to see a 5-year income statement. In addition, in this case, notice that under operational expenses, there is a line item named "debt service." This is the monthly payment to be made to an investor who loaned the company its start-up capital. The monthly payment includes principal and interest at 9% amortized over a 5-year period.

OPERATIONAL EXPENSES

	Dec-10	Jan-11	Feb-11	Mar-11	Apr-11	May-11	Jun-11	Jul-11	Aug-11	Sep-11	Oct-11	Nov-11	Dec-11	FYE 12.31.11
Rent		3,000	3,000	3,000	3,000	3,000	3,000	3,000	3,000	3,000	3,000	3,000	3,000	36,000
Marketing		2,160	2,160	2,160	2,160	2,160	2,160	2,160	2,160	2,160	2,160	2,160	2,160	25,915
Office Supplies		50	75	200	100	100	200	100	100	250	150	150	200	1,675
Uniforms			150		150				150		150			600
Water / fruit														
Postage		3	5	2,107	9	12	14	16	2,167	20	22	24	26	4,426
Cable / Internet / Telephone		200	200	200	200	200	200	200	200	200	200	200	200	2,400
Biz Insurance		350	350	350	350	350	350	350	350	350	350	350	350	4,200
Insurance — GL&U		338	338	338	338	338	338	338	338	338	338	338	338	4,051
Insurance — Workers Comp		150	150	150	150	150	150	150	150	150	150	150	150	1,800
Maintenance / laundry														
Insurance														
Banking / Credit Card fees		262	321	380	438	512	559	617	676	747	806	865	924	7,106
Debt Service *($108,367 5 yr @ 9%)*		2,250	2,250	2,250	2,250	2,250	2,250	2,250	2,250	2,250	2,250	2,250	2,250	27,000
		8,762	8,998	11,134	9,145	9,070	9,219	9,180	11,541	9,464	9,575	9,486	9,597	115,172
DIRECT EXPENSES														
Mgr's salary *(75,000)*	6,250	6,250	6,250	6,250	6,250	6,250	6,250	6,250	6,250	6,250	6,250	6,250	6,250	75,000
Payroll taxes *(7,500)*		625	625	625	625	625	625	625	625	625	625	625	625	7,500
Health Benefits *(9,000)*		750	750	750	750	750	750	750	750	750	750	750	750	9,000
Professional Dues / Travel				524					1,500		1,500			3,524
Trainers' pay			1,766	2,472	4,259	5,205	6,152	7,098	9,005	10,065	11,866	12,996	14,126	85,010
Trainers' p/r taxes			177	247	426	521	615	710	901	1,006	1,187	1,300	1,413	8,501
Benefits						521	615	710	901	1,006	1,187	1,300	1,413	7,651
Group Instructor's pay		1,400	1,400	1,400	1,400	1,400	800	800	800	1,400	1,400	1,400	1,400	15,000
Trainers' p/r taxes		140	140	140	140	140	80	80	80	140	140	140	140	1,500
Benefits														
	6,250	9,165	11,107	12,408	13,850	15,412	15,887	17,023	20,811	21,243	24,904	24,760	26,116	212,687
TOTAL EXPENSES	6,250	17,927	20,106	23,542	22,995	24,482	25,107	26,203	32,352	30,707	34,479	34,246	35,713	327,859
INCOME														
PT Revenue		4,238	7,063	9,888	12,713	15,539	18,364	21,189	24,014	26,839	29,665	32,490	35,315	237,317
Ave #/wkly client-hrs		15	25	35	45	55	65	75	85	95	105	115	125	125
# of client-hours		60	100	140	180	220	260	300	340	380	420	460	500	500
$ per session		70.63	70.63	70.63	70.63	70.63	70.63	70.63	70.63	70.63	70.63	70.63	70.63	70.63
Bootcamps Revenue *($1695/24 sessions)*		3,456	3,456	3,456	3,456	3,456	2,880	2,880	2,880	3,456	3,456	3,456	3,456	39,744
Ave #/classes per week		9	9	9	9	9	6	6	6	9	9	9	9	9
Ave #/clients per class		8	8	8	8	8	10	10	10	8	8	8	8	8
Ave #/wkly client-hours		72	72	72	72	72	60	60	60	72	72	72	72	72
# of clients-hours		288	288	288	288	288	240	240	240	288	288	288	288	288
$ per client-hour *(80%/$150/10 sessions)*		12.00	12.00	12.00	12.00	12.00	12.00	12.00	12.00	12.00	12.00	12.00	12.00	12.00
insPIRE Baseball Conditioning Revenue		3,446	3,446	3,446	3,446	4,136	4,136	4,136	4,136	4,136	4,136	4,136	4,136	46,871
Ave #/classes per week		8	8	8	8	8	8	8	8	8	8	8	8	8
Ave #/clients per class		5	5	5	5	6	6	6	6	6	6	6	6	6
Ave #/wkly client-hours		40	40	40	40	48	48	48	48	48	48	48	48	48
# of clients-hours		160	160	160	160	192	192	192	192	192	192	192	192	192
$ per client-hour *(80%/$350/13 sessions)*		21.54	21.54	21.54	21.54	21.54	21.54	21.54	21.54	21.54	21.54	21.54	21.54	21.54
TOTAL INCOME	-	11,140	13,965	16,791	19,616	23,130	25,379	28,205	31,030	34,431	37,256	40,081	42,907	323,932
EBITDA =	(6,250)	(6,787)	(6,140)	(6,752)	(3,379)	(1,352)	273	2,001	(1,322)	3,724	2,777	5,835	7,194	(3,927)
Accumulated net =	(6,250.00)	(6,787.07)	(12,927.21)	(19,679.01)	(23,058.17)	(24,409.78)	(24,136.85)	(22,135.39)	(23,457.65)	(19,733.41)	(16,956.18)	(11,120.77)	(3,927.21)	

Direct-expense annual references (gray boxes): 75,000 / 7,500 / 9,000. PT income note: staff trainers / sess/wk.

Figure 12-2. First year Operating Budget for Sports Training Academy

Once the fiscal month has passed and the budget is reconciled with the actual expense and income numbers of the business during that month, it will serve as an "Actuals" budget or simply the business's P&L statement for that period. Any profits or losses are expressed in the form of earnings before income taxes, depreciation, and amortization (EBITDA). EBITDA is equal to the gross margin (the difference between total sales revenue and total direct cost of sales) minus total operating expenses (tax-deductible expenses incurred in conducting normal business operations, such as wages and salaries, rent, etc.), plus any depreciation (the loss of value of assets over time) and amortization.

Once again, it is important to note that unless you have extensive expertise in preparing financial statements, start-up budgets, P&Ls, and cash-flow statements should really be left to an accounting professional. Chapter 13, Selling Your Dream, will focus on using the business plan and financial statements to raise and secure capital for the launch of the business. It will be imperative that management and investors be able to fully understand every number on every financial statement in the plan. Management's passion and confidence have to show through when presenting the business plan to prospective investors.

CHAPTER SUMMARY

The most basic financial statements in a business plan include the start-up budget, operating budget/income statement, and cash-flow statement. These are simple documents that the business owner/operator will use to effectively manage the business. However, during the development of the initial financial statements for the business, the help of an accounting or bookkeeping professional is paramount to ensuring accurate, realistic, and appropriate financial projections and reporting.

YOUR RESOURCES

U.S. Small Business Administration, as seen at: http://www.sba.gov/smallbusinessplanner/plan/writeabusinessplan/serv_bp_financials.html

REFERENCES

1. IRS gov, Small Businesses, 2011. [cited 2011 August 21]. Available from: http://www.irs.gov/businesses/small/article/0,id=137026,00.html

13 Selling Your Dream

Chapter Objectives

After reading this chapter, the reader will:

- Understand some of the basic steps of making a formal request for funding
- Know some of the more common ways (*i.e.*, debt, equity) to fund a new business enterprise
- Be aware of the U.S. Small Business Association (SBA) and how they can assist an entrepreneur in the process of funding their business.

FINANCING THE PROJECT

So now that the business plan is complete with marketing plan and financial statements, it's time to either write a check to fund the business or acquire the funds necessary for a successful launch of the business. It is not too often that entrepreneurs reach into their own pockets to fully fund a project. More often than not, the prospective business owner must go out and look to either a bank or private equity investor for the start-up capital for their business.

DEBT

One funding possibility is acquiring a loan or using a credit line to fund the project. Depending on how much capital is needed to launch the business, this could mean simply reaching into one's own pocket for credit cards, or perhaps a credit line based on the equity of the entrepreneur's home. In most cases, entrepreneurs will apply for a business loan through their bank, or making a fund request via the U.S. Small Business Association (SBA), an independent agency of the federal government whose mission is to aid, counsel, assist, and protect the interests of small businesses.

The SBA can be very helpful to the entrepreneur throughout the financing process, because it will help point the entrepreneur in the right direction throughout the process. Entrepreneurs will follow a streamlined process requesting the amount of funding they will need to start or expand their business. They can include different funding scenarios, such as a best- and worst-case scenario, keeping in mind that later, in the financial section of their funding request, they must be able to back up these requests and scenarios with corresponding financial statements.

Entrepreneurs will provide their current funding requirement, their future funding requirements over the next 5 years, how they will use the funds they receive, and any long-range financial strategies that they are planning that would have any type of impact on their funding request. They would include the amount they want now and the amount they want in the future, the time period that each request will cover, the type of funding they would like to have (*i.e.*, equity, debt), and the terms that they would like to have applied. How they will use the funds is very important to a creditor. Is the funding request for capital expenditures, working capital, debt retirement, or acquisitions?

Entrepreneurs are also prompted to include any strategic information related to their business that may have an impact on their financial situation in the future, such as going public with their company, having a leveraged buyout, being acquired by another company, the method with which they will service their debt, or whether or not they plan to sell their business in the future. Each of these is extremely important to a future creditor, since they will directly impact the business owner's ability to repay the loan(s) (1).

EQUITY FINANCING

Equity financing involves the sale of some portion of ownership in a venture to gain additional capital for start-up. For example, the entrepreneur might have $30,000 to invest in the business but need $100,000 to launch it. He or she can pitch the business venture to a private investor who will provide the $70,000 needed for start-up. In return for the investment, the entrepreneur receives a negotiated share of the business. He or she might start with a 70% equity position, and as management works and builds the business, it earns "sweat equity" until each owns 50%. This is a simplified illustration of how to develop an equity agreement with an investor. It can certainly be much more complicated, but the premise is the same. The investor will provide money in return for a portion of the business.

THE PITCH

Whether management pursues funding at the local commercial bank, goes through the SBA, or finds an interested private investor, it must put its best foot forward when presenting the opportunity that the business represents.

Use your network of colleagues and other professionals in the industry to "spread the word" of the venture and find private financing. Answer every query, and identify qualified private investors. Prepare a document that includes the business plan's executive summary, and a one-page 5-year financial summary or pro forma (projected profit and loss, P&L) statement. Use this document to cultivate interest in the business venture. When you find a real prospective investor, schedule a sit-down meeting with them so you can present a complete business plan to them (Box 13.1).

BOX 13.1	**GIVE INVESTORS A WAY OUT!**
	It is important when painting the picture of the business plan for a prospective investor that it includes an exit strategy that the investor might use at some point in order to "collect" the return on his or her investment and be "off the hook." Common exit strategies include a management buyout or an initial public offering. The exit strategy will be dependent on the size and scope of your business plan. Unless the business is large enough to attract the assistance of an investment house that will "take you public," a management buyout is likely to be your most feasible exit strategy. This could require planning on management's part so that it is able at a predetermined point in time to buy out the investor with funds it has saved, credit from a bank, or other lender, or it can find other investors who will fund the continued growth of the business as well as buy out the initial investor(s).

PRESENTING THE PLAN

When presenting the business plan to an investor, it is wise to use and have the investor sign a nondisclosure agreement, which binds the investor to keep private any information shared with him or her. Number the investor's copy of the business plan and write the corresponding number on the nondisclosure agreement. This will help keep track of the distributed copies of the business plan.

Remember that a picture is worth a thousand words. Streamline the business plan by developing a PowerPoint presentation that highlights the major points of the business plan. This will keep the presentation on task and keep the investor listening instead of reading the in-depth plan or financials while you are explaining your marketing strategy or describing your management team. After the presentation, the investor will take the complete business plan with him or her and will be able to review it in its entirety.

At the end of the Triad Fitness business plan on page 202 you will find a brief presentation that highlights the major selling points of the Triad business plan. This presentation is included in this book in grayscale. It is recommended to use bright colors and graphics in your presentation to make it visually appealing. Depending on how and where you present your plan, you can project the plan on a video screen, have it loaded on a laptop to present it live at a table at the local coffee house, or print out a hard-copy for your prospective investor to page through as you present it.

PLANNING AHEAD
There is a sample business plan presentation for Triad Fitness on page 202.

CHAPTER SUMMARY

There are very basic steps to requesting funding for your business venture. The most common ways to finance your venture are either debt financing or equity financing. Debt financing is essentially a loan that is paid back in principal and interest. Equity financing involves selling or providing ownership for a portion of your business to the investor. A formal request for funding may be submitted via the U.S. SBA, whose mission is to help the small business owner succeed over the long haul.

YOUR RESOURCES

U.S. Small Business Association
http://www.sba.gov/

Business.gov — helps small businesses understand their legal requirements and locate government services from federal, state, and local agencies.
http://www.business.gov/

The Association of Small Business Development Centers (ASBDC) represents America's Small Business Development Center Network, the most comprehensive small business assistance network in the United States and its territories. The mission of the network is to help new entrepreneurs realize the dream of business ownership, and to assist existing businesses to remain competitive in the complex marketplace of an ever-changing global economy. Hosted by leading universities, colleges, and state economic development agencies, and funded in part through a partnership with the U.S. Small Business Administration, approximately 1,000 service centers are available to provide no-cost consulting and low-cost training. To find a Small Business Development Center near you, go to http://www.asbdc-us.org/ and search by your zip code or your state in the light blue box on the right side of the web page.

REFERENCES

1. U.S. Small Business Administration. Loans, 2011 [cited 2011 August 21]. Available from: http://www.sba.gov/category/navigation-structure/starting-managing-business/starting-business/loans-grants-funding/loans

3

Business Plan, Budgets, and Presentation

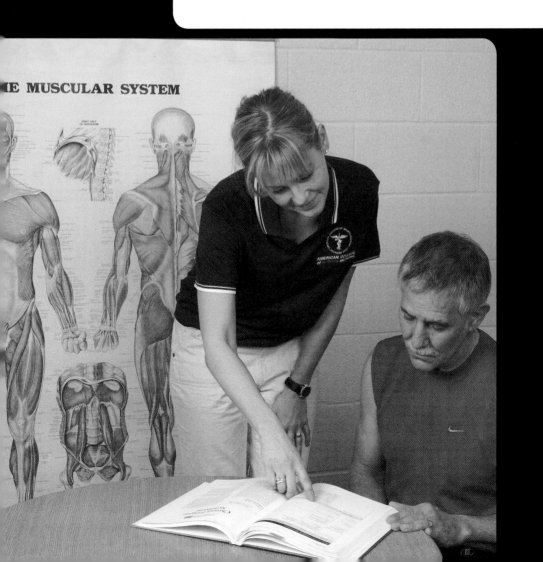

Business Plan

Triad Fitness

Health, Performance, and Fitness
for the Entire Family

ABC FITNESS CORPORATION
DBA TRIAD FITNESS
CONTENTS

I. EXECUTIVE SUMMARY

The Purpose of this Business Plan is to arrange for start-up capital along with working capital for a series of Triad-branded premium physical fitness programs, products, and services (The Company) to meet the fitness needs and active lifestyles of our proposed members. The total initial capital required will be $2,125,000. This money will be used to design, construct, and equip the center as well as provide the necessary start-up and working capital.

The Company is seeking its funding of $2,125,000 through private investment for either an equity position in the Company or a loan to the Company with an appropriate interest rate to be paid by the Company.

The Products and Services of the Company will consist of an adult physical fitness program (Adult Physical Fitness Program at Triad Fitness, APFP) and two children's programs (the Athlete Training Center at Triad Fitness [ATC] and the Youth Fitness Zone at Triad Fitness [YFZ]). The APFP will be an upgraded version of Physiofitness Center, which was a New York–based, successful, medically oriented, supervised, and individualized exercise program designed to help its members take an active role in their preventive health care. Triad plans on providing an exceptional member experience to inspire and motivate its members to achieve results within a facility of quality and innovative design. The two children's programs will be an athletic conditioning program called the ATC, which is devoted to helping athletes in every sport, at all ages, and all skill levels realize their athletic potential through advanced sports performance training programs, and a children's remedial physical fitness program called the YFZ for the deconditioned and for the obese youth market, which has recently received a good deal of media attention with respect to the federal government's concern for this important and sometimes overlooked population.

All our members will enjoy the benefits of our emphasis on service, value, quality, expertise, innovation of programs, and attention to detail. We will encourage our members to participate in our programs and services and to use our facilities frequently. We believe that participating members will get results and will be more likely to renew their memberships and to refer new members. Participating members are also more likely to use high-margin ancillary programs and services, such as personal training and nutrition services.

The Size and Location The first proposed training facility will consist of approximately 17,500 sq ft and is anticipated to be located in Allendale, New Jersey, which clearly meets our demographic criteria within one of the most affluent counties in New Jersey. Operating in the middle to upper end market segment of the fragmented fitness industry, we target an attractive demographic member profile. Our typical member is a well-educated professional between 25 and 65 years of age with significant discretionary income and who considers fitness an essential part of his or her active lifestyle.

This proposed location gives the best visibility of the facility from Route 17 South. The space rental rates are a bit more than other spaces that management has seen, but it believes it is worth paying a premium for this location, because of its visibility from Route 17 South. It should be noted here that the APFP will have its own separate facilities within the scope of the entire facility consisting of approximately ten thousand square feet (10,000 sq ft) and the two other programs will share approximately seven thousand five hundred square feet (7,500 sq ft).

The Management Team of Triad Fitness has the vision, experience, and passion to successfully manage growth and will consist of the following three professionals:

> William T. Smith was co-founder and former President of Physiofitness Corporation, Inc., an operator of upscale, medically-oriented physical fitness centers in New York City, Chicago and Toronto, Canada. Mr. Smith was responsible, along with his partners, for growing the business and selling it to XYZ Holdings, Inc. in 1985. It is anticipated that Mr. Smith will be the President and Chief Executive Officer of the Company and will be responsible for the Company's day-to-day operations and administration as well as managing the sales process of the company.
>
> Carlo I. Pirelli developed a very successful prototype of the Company's proposed Children's Programs for a fitness company based in Northern New Jersey. It is anticipated that Mr. Pirelli will be an Executive Vice President of the Company and Director of the all the Children's Programs.
>
> Thomas Milkin is the owner of Fitness-4-U, a one on one personal training studio for adults located in Waldwick, NJ. Mr. Milkin has had extensive experience in working with adults of the same socioeconomic profile as the target market of the Company. It is anticipated that Mr. Milkin will be an Executive Vice President of the Company and Director of the Adult Physical Fitness Programs.

The Adult Physical Fitness Program will be managed by Mr. Milkin. It will be an improved modification of the aforementioned successful Physiofitness Program, which had a proven record of membership sales similar to the demographics of Allendale, New Jersey. This Business Plan has taken a more conservative monthly membership sales rate (average of 50 new member sales per month) than the rates achieved by the Physiofitness Company and those of competitors within the Allendale, New Jersey area (Physiofitness monthly new member sales average = 75 to 90, competitors' monthly new member sales average = 110 to 150).

The Athlete Training Center will be headed by Mr. Pirelli who has had extensive experience in the management of these types of training programs. His experience indicates that monthly sales revenues in a similar-size training facility in a community within Bergen County, New Jersey, (not within Triad's immediate marketing area) are approximately $65,000. Carlo has taken a very conservative approach in forecasting the monthly sales of ATC, using an average of $32,400. Within a 15-mile radius of Allendale, New Jersey, there are approximately 300,000 children who represent the potential market base for this program. Mr. Pirelli has an excellent relationship with many of the coaches (covering all sports) within Bergen County. The ATC program will be marketed to these coaches in several different ways; it will also be marketed to pediatricians in the area as well as via an aggressive advertising campaign will be developed for the parents of these athletes.

The Youth Fitness Zone will be a unique and very exciting aspect of the Company's offerings. The deconditioned and often obese youth market has mushroomed within the United States in the past several years. Latest statistics indicate that 15% of children and adolescents are either overweight or obese, with another 15% designated "at risk" (CDC 2000). This represents a significant segment of the youth population in the United States. Within a 15-mile radius of Allendale, New Jersey, there are approximately 100,000 children who represent the potential, untapped market base for this program. As of this date, there are no private firms in the proposed demographic area (and for that matter within the United States) marketing this type of programming to the parents of deconditioned and usually obese children. If Triad gets its funding and develops its programs at the proposed Allendale location, this should preempt any competition that may develop.

The Surgeon General's Call to Action 2001 Report points to the lack of physical activity as a major contributor to this effect. The recommendations for children from this report are

- Reduce TV watching time.
- Promote healthier food choices at home, school, and aftercare.
- Ensure that children get 60 minutes of moderate activity most days of the week.

It is unfortunate that the public school systems within the United States either do not put enough emphasis on the values of the Physical Education Program or just do not have enough money in their school budgets to support this program.

The Company will retain an experienced advertising agency that has done the advertising for the Physiofitness Centers when they were owned by

Mr. Smith and his partners. They will differentiate the Company's services and programs from the "typical health club" market through aggressive, sophisticated, targeted advertising and marketing, which will carve out the Company's market niche in this affluent area in New Jersey.

The exceptional talents and experience of its Management Team will play an extremely important role in the company's success. The proprietary systems for the services and products being offered, the chosen location, the demographics of its target market and the experience of the advertising agency are all very important to the success of the Company, but the quality, experience, and dedication of its management team will be the intangible assets that make this business successful.

It is the intent of the management team to open three more of these facilities within the next 5 years within the New York metropolitan area. The Company anticipates using internal funding for its expansion plans. Management believes that there is a possibility of franchising parts or all of the Company's various services.

Management also believes that an exit strategy for an equity investor might well be selling the Company to a larger national or international fitness firm, a firm in a related health care industry, a management buyout, or for the Company to do an Initial Public Offering. Management also believes another exit strategy might be selling each mature facility to the landlord of the center with Triad receiving a long-term management contract, which will have a performance bonus associated with it.

Financial Data Analysis: As can be determined by the following financial information, the management expects to be at break even on an "Earnings Before Interest, Taxes, Depreciation and Amortization" (EBITDA) basis by the end of year 1.

Business Objectives

- To acquire 600+ adult memberships by end of the first year of operation
- To exceed 50% ATC session capacity by the end of the first year of operation
- Achieve breakeven on an EBITDA basis by the end of year 1

Mission

Triad Fitness' mission is to create a family-oriented workout environment that promotes self-confidence in our clients in playing a proactive role in the prevention of chronic disease through physical activity and healthy lifestyle.

FIVE-YEAR PROJECTIONS OF EBIDTA

	Year 1(*) C: 1	% of Revenue	Year 2 C: 1	% of Revenue	Year 3 C: 1 & 2	% of Revenue	Year 4 C: 1, 2, & 3	% of Revenue	Year 5 C: 1, 2, 3, & 4	% of Revenue
Total Revenue	$1,526,889	100%	$2,746,531	100%	$5,525,079	100%	$8,906,555	100%	$13,332,866	100%
Total Direct Expenses	$950,304	62.23%	$1,401,351	51.02%	$2,530,707	46.80%	$3,756,047	42.17%	$5,386,168	40.04%
Total Operating Expenses	$535,132	35.05%	$686,242	24.99%	$1,362,488	24.66%	$2,119,180	23.79%	$2,988,453	22.412%
Operating Profit	$41,453	2.71%	$658,938	23.99%	$1,631,884	29.54%	$3,031,329	34.03%	$4,958,245	37.19%
Employee Bonus	$0	$0	$65,894	2.39%	$152,583	2.76%	$283,016	3.18%	$473,818	3.55%
Employee Taxes & Benefits @ 25%	$0	$0	$16,473	0.60%	$38,146	0.69%	$70,754	0.79%	$118,455	0.89%
EBITDA	$41,453	2.71%	$576,571	20.99%	$1,441,155	26.08%	$2,677,559	30.06%	$4,365,972	32.75%

*(C), Center(s) number.

Company Summary

Triad Fitness is a fitness club that offers medically oriented exercise training, fitness classes, a performance training program for adolescent athletes, and a unique fitness program for otherwise inactive children with a focus on servicing the obese child. William T. Smith will oversee all business operations. Carlo I. Pirelli will manage both the ATC and the YFZ, and Thomas Milkin will manage the APFP.

II. OVERVIEW

The Fitness and Health Club Industry

The Fitness industry growth patterns and demographics present an attractive business environment, particularly in the middle to high-end niche that Triad targets. The fitness industry includes commercial facilities, YMCA facilities, nonprofit facilities, gyms, hospital-operated facilities, and country clubs. Total industry revenues in 2002 were approximately $13.1 billion.

The fitness and health club industry is a highly fragmented industry that has grown significantly in the past 2 decades as the public has become increasingly aware of the benefits of regular exercise and an improved level of physical fitness. As of December 31, 2002, there were 20,249 health clubs listed in various business databases, which is a 14% growth rate over 2001. The number of health clubs has increased consistently over the past 5 years, up 44% from 14,100 businesses in 1998. Consumer demand for health clubs remained strong in 2002, growing from 33.8 million members in 2001 to 36.3 million members in 2002 — a 7.5% increase, despite the poor economy.

On July 11, 1996, the Surgeon General of the United States released the "Surgeon General's Report on Physical Activity and Health" (Exhibit A). This report indicated that "lack of regular exercise is associated with premature death and increased coronary risk profiles for heart disease, type 2 diabetes, osteoporosis, and some forms of cancer." It also stated that "regular exercise lowers resting heart rates, reduces cholesterol, increases HDL and lowers LDL, and is a major factor in weight management. Also regular exercise promotes healthy sleep patterns, reduces anxiety and depression, and preserves sex drive, strength, and mobility into old age."

These proven health benefits of exercise have spurred older Americans to join health clubs. An International Health, Racquet and Sportsclub Association/ American Sports Data, Inc. Health Club Trend Report states that "from 1955 to 2001, the percentage of health club members age 55 and over grew by 68%. And since the release of the Surgeon General's Report, there also has been a shift in the age demographics of health clubs, with older members accounting for a significantly greater percentage of members."

The Surgeon General's office gave a further boost to the health club industry with their December 13, 2001, release of The Surgeon General's Call to Action to Prevent and Decrease Overweight and Obesity (Exhibit B). This document indicated that being obese or even being 10 pounds overweight was associated with premature death, heart disease, cancer, depression, and more than a dozen other diseases and disorders. Their recommendations stated that we must "Ensure that adults get 30 minutes of moderate activity on most days."

The report indicated that "for the vast majority of individuals, overweight and obesity result from excess calorie consumption and/or inadequate physical activity." It also stated that "as of January 1, 2000, 61% (approximately 122 million) of American adults were classified as being either overweight or obese; of these, 54 million were classified as clinically obese and 68 million were classified as overweight or pre-obese."

More recently in 2001, the Surgeon General's Office reported that "Since 1980 the number of children who are overweight has doubled and the number of overweight adolescents has tripled."

Given the above figures on the adult population and statements made by the Surgeon General's Office on children's obesity, this would lead one to conclude that, following the 1996 Surgeon General's Report and its 2001 Call to Action to Prevent and Decrease Overweight and Obesity, health clubs can expect the acceleration in membership growth to continue. Therefore, management believes it can capture this high growth potential in this fragmented industry with the Company's focused approach of services and products to the selected demographic population.

The Company

The Company (Triad Fitness) will be a premium provider of an adult physical fitness program (APFP) and two children's programs (the ATC and the YFZ). The APFP) will be an upgraded version of Physiofitness Center, which was a successful, medically oriented, supervised, and individualized exercise program to help the members take an active role in their preventive health care. Triad plans on providing an exceptional member experience to inspire and motivate its members to achieve results within a facility of quality and innovative design. The two children's programs will be an athletic conditioning program called the ATC, which is devoted to helping athletes in every sport, at all ages, and all skill levels realize their athletic potential through advanced sports performance training programs, and a children's remedial physical fitness program called the YFZ for the deconditioned and for the most part obese youth market, which has recently received a good deal of media attention with respect to the federal government's concern for this important and sometimes overlooked population.

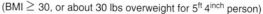

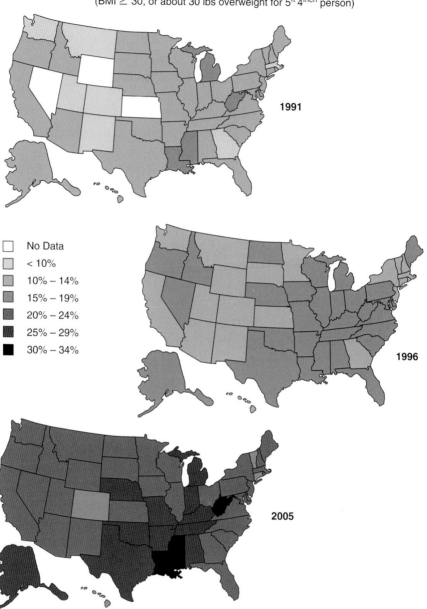

Obesity trends among US adults. Courtesy of Centers for Disease Control and Prevention.

The first facility is anticipated to be located in Allendale, New Jersey, which is one of the most affluent counties and residential areas in New Jersey. The Company will have an excellent chance of success largely due to the exceptional talents, experience, and dedication of its management team as well as factors such as its marketing and advertising plan, location of the facility, demographics of its target market, and the unique products and services it offers.

III.   MANAGEMENT

Led by our President and CEO, William T. Smith, we believe our management team has the vision, experience, and passion to manage our envisioned growth.

William T. Smith is former Chief Operating Officer of VIP Health Management, Inc., a leading provider of supervised, medically based Adult Physical Fitness Programs, Physical Therapy Clinics, and Spa/Massage Services in New York City, New Jersey, Chicago, Ohio, and California. He spearheaded VIP Health Management's growth from 1994 doing $3.5 MM in sales to 2003 with a Fiscal Year Ending (FYE) projection of $18.75 MM in sales. He was cofounder and former President of Physiofitness Corporation, Inc., an operator of upscale, medically oriented physical fitness centers in New York City, Chicago, and Toronto, Canada. He was responsible, along with his partners, for growing the business and selling it to XYZ Holdings, Inc. in 1985. Prior to that in 1971, he created (the first of its kind in the United States) a medically based "in-house" Executive Physical Fitness Program for U.S. National Oil Corp. He received his Master of Science degree in Exercise Physiology with a concentration in Cardiac Rehabilitation from Adirondack College. It is anticipated that he will be the President and Chief Executive Officer of the Company and will be responsible for the Company's day-to-day administration.

Carlo I. Pirelli has been a professional in the commercial fitness industry for the past 24 years and is currently Director of Training at VIP Health Management, Inc. As part of VIP Health Management's Senior Management Team, he has developed innovative systems and protocols that have optimized customer service and fitness training services. He has also developed one of the most comprehensive initial and continuing education programs in the industry for the company's estimated 250 exercise specialists. Prior to joining VIP Health Management, Inc., he developed the successful prototype of the Company's proposed Children's Programs for a fitness company based in northern New Jersey. He also serves on several national and international committees and special interest groups on behalf of ACSM, the American Council on Exercise, and the National Strength and Conditioning Association (NSCA). In addition, he has strong entrepreneurial ambitions coupled with the ability to work long hours. He earned a Master's degree in Exercise Physiology from Ivy University.

It is anticipated that he will be an Executive Vice President of the Company and Director of the all the Children's Programs.

Thomas Milkin is the owner of Fitness-4-U, a one-on-one personal training studio located in Waldwick, New Jersey. As you can see by his ownership of his own business, he has strong entrepreneurial desires coupled with the ability to work long hours. Prior to starting his own business, he worked at VIP Health Management, Inc. as Assistant Manager at their World Trade Center and Director of Personal Training for VIP Health Management's Wall Street account. During his tenure at Wall Street, he increased personal training revenue by 72%. He was the fitness director for Ellen Sailor Hospital in Cranston, Rhode Island, where he was responsible for developing the fitness-based testing protocol for all of the mentally challenged, paraplegic, and quadriplegic patients, which is still being used today. He also served as the Fitness Director for the United States Naval Academy in Providence, Rhode Island, where he was nationally recognized for designing the base's new 40,000 sq ft fitness facility. He holds a Master of Science degree in Exercise Physiology from the University of New England. It is anticipated that he will be an Executive Vice President of the Company and Director of the APFP.

IV.   DEPARTMENTS AND CONCEPTS

Adult Physical Fitness

The Company's business strategy for the APFP is to appeal to a primary target market of mature, affluent, well-educated, physically deconditioned, overweight men and women 35 years and older. This market values personal service, professionally trained staff, as well as safe, customized, and goal-oriented programs of physical fitness. This facility will not be your typical health club. It will be an upscale exercise facility professionally designed for busy people who wish to get in shape and stay in shape in a more time-efficient and controlled manner than the standard health club can provide. The Company's policy of limiting membership of each gender based on maximum capacity that the facility can accommodate will ensure that our members will not be inconvenienced in having to wait to use our exercise equipment or any of our support facilities. This program is not about pumping up pecs or parading around in fancy workout clothes, but improving levels of physical fitness and controlling coronary risk factors so our members feel better, look better, and perform better. The individual programs developed for members will adhere to the highest professional standards, including the recommendations and guidelines set forth by the American Heart Association, the American Medical Association, and the ACSM for the middle-aged, deconditioned population.

A prospective member of APFP must complete a Physical Activity Readiness Questionnaire (PARQ). If the prospective member answers yes to any of the PARQ questions and their existing coronary risk profile puts them into the ACSM "moderate risk level," he or she must have their personal physician complete a Medical History Form signed by the doctor and sent to the general manager of the center. It will be the general manager's responsibility to review the Medical History Form and determine if the Company's APFP is right for this prospective member, or if he or she needs a cardiac or physical rehabilitation program before they start with the Company's APFP. Once the prospective member becomes a member of the Company's APFP, their physical fitness level is established by using a variety of physiological (*i.e.*, physical work capacity test), body composition, strength, and flexibility tests. Along with the results of these tests and an interview with the member to determine his or her personal goals, a custom-tailored, goal-oriented, individual exercise program will be developed for each member (to do within our center). The results of these physical fitness tests will be printed in a quality form and presented to the member for his or her use.

The management has developed several successful, proprietary program features in order to keep our members motivated and interested to keep coming into the center to exercise. These include at least one exercise physiologist will visit each member during his or her exercise session to discuss the exercise program, and take his or her heart rate and or blood pressure. Also, each time a person exercises within our center and completes their exercise program for the day, an exercise physiologist will review their exercise program card and develop a new (if appropriate) series of exercise program goals to be completed on their next visit to the center. Therefore, each member will receive their updated, individualized, safe, and goal-oriented exercise program(s) to be completed within the Company's facilities. In addition, the APFP will feature a well-defined and established program to assure member attendance. Each member will be assigned a personal exercise physiologist (PEP) who will track his or her performance and attendance to the center. If the member does not use the Center within a 2-week period, the PEP will call him or her in order to set up a time for the member's return to exercise.

The fact that the Company's strategy is to establish its offerings as a family-oriented fitness center broadens its appeal and reach into the community. The Adult Physical Fitness Department will become a "feeder program" for the other programs offered by the Company. It is management's assumption that the APFP members will refer their children to the Company's ATC or its YFZ.

Sports Training Center

The ATC will be another offering of the Company that is devoted to helping athletes in every sport, at all ages, and all skill levels realize their athletic potential through advanced sports performance training programs. The potential member of this program will go through a set of physical performance assessments in order to determine that the athlete has the baseline physical fitness level and skill level required to participate in the training program. Assessment results may indicate that the individual does not have the prerequisite abilities to participate in the ATC program and will benefit from enrolling in the YFZ program. In such cases, the program director will discuss these findings with the child's parents and make the appropriate recommendations. If the child has the prerequisite fitness and skill levels required to participate in the program, the program director will then develop an appropriate training protocol based on the athlete's current abilities, the physical requirements of their sport, and their personal sports-related goals. The training will be done within the Company's facility.

The programs will be scientifically designed to maximize the individual's sports performance. The strategic approach to ATC is that professional and amateur sports are becoming increasingly competitive (these athletes need a "competitive edge"), a trend, that is prompting parents to seek out ways to improve their child's performance and abilities. At the same time, school budgets are being cut and fewer resources are available for sports conditioning programs. Consequently, school districts are looking for partners within the community to help fill the void. The ATC director will work very closely with school administrators and coaches to support their programs and goals. The ATC director will also market the Company's Team Camps and Coaches' Clinics, which will extend its reach out into the sports training community, expanding its brand name and market share. The Company's management will also position itself as a leader amongst its peers by presenting at coaches' conferences on a regional and national level.

Therefore, the target market for the Company's ATC will be student athletes aged 8–20, recreational athletes, elite amateur athletes, and professional athletes. Within a 15-mile radius of Allendale, New Jersey, there are approximately 300,000 children who represent the potential market base for this program. The fact that the Company's strategy is to establish its offerings to be a family-oriented fitness center broadens its appeal and reach into the community. The ATC department will become a "feeder program" for the APFP and YFZ programs.

While the Company's management believes youth sports conditioning is in its infancy and expects other entities to mimic its operation in the future, management is taking maximum advantage of the current market conditions to solidify its position as the category leader creating national brand recognition.

Youth Fitness Zone

The YFZ will be a unique and very exciting aspect of the Company's offerings. The deconditioned and usually obese youth market has mushroomed within the United States in the past several years. Latest statistics indicate that

15% of children and adolescents are either overweight or obese, with another 15% designated "at risk" (CDC 2000). This represents a significant segment of the youth population in the United States. Within a 15-mile radius of Allendale, New Jersey, there are approximately 100,000 children who represent the potential, untapped market base for this program. As of this date, there are no private firms in the proposed demographic area (and for that matter within the United States) marketing this type of programming to the parents of deconditioned and usually obese children. If Triad gets its funding and develops its programs, our presence should preempt any competition that may develop.

The Surgeon General's Call to Action 2001 Report points to the lack of physical activity as a major contributor to this effect. The recommendations for children from this report are

- Reduce TV watching time.
- Promote healthier food choices at home, school, and aftercare.
- Ensure that children get 60 minutes of moderate activity most days of the week.

It is unfortunate that the public school systems within the United States either do not put enough emphasis on the values of the Physical Education Program or just do not have enough money in their school budgets to support this program. The Sporting Goods Manufacturers Association reports that:

- 1991 — 81% of enrolled students were active for at least 20 minutes.
- 1995 — 70% were active.
- Currently, fewer than 25% are active.

Through its relationship with the local schools, the local area pediatricians, and community(s) at large, the Company will target this group and provide a basic conditioning module (to be completed within the Company's center) that will address their needs. This program will further solidify the Company's presence as an "expert" in youth fitness, while broadening its appeal to the community. As of this date, there are no private firms in the proposed demographic area (and for that matter within the United States) marketing this type of programming to the parents of deconditioned and usually obese children, which should preempt any competition that may develop.

Ancillary Services

We believe we will set the industry standard of excellence with our quality and innovative programming. We believe that a member's experience and loyalty is driven by the results achieved through their personal exercise programs, service, and attention to detail. We will offer additional ancillary programming, such as personal training, and nutritional services on a fee-for-service basis, thereby generating revenues.

Personal Training

We believe personal training is one of the most effective ways to help our members reach their health and fitness goals. All exercise physiologists will be instructed to cross-sell all our offerings, including personal training packages and other services that will help the member achieve his or her goals. Our personal training will be customized to the needs of each member within our proprietary training methodology and system. The personal training pricing is structured to appeal to the widest demographic of the center. We will offer various packages with the price dependent upon the number of sessions purchased.

Nutrition Programs

Working with a registered dietitian our members can purchase an advanced nutrition analysis and weight management program developed for optimal health. The registered dietitian will guide the member through a 6-week program specifically designed to get results and provide the member with the knowledge and guidance needed to make changes in their nutrition profile that will work and last.

V.   STAFFING

The Company's success will depend in large part on the quality of the staff management recruits and trains. The Company will staff each program with professional exercise physiologists who have a minimum of a Bachelor of Science or Arts in such areas as Exercise Physiology, Cardiac Rehabilitation, Athletic Training, Adult Physical Fitness, or Physical Education. Each staff member will be certified by the ACSM as a health fitness instructor and/or the NSCA, and will be certified in cardiopulmonary resuscitation by either the American Heart Association or The American Red Cross.

Management will also look for an overall professionalism in the prospective exercise physiologists. They must be pleasant, helpful, enthusiastic, and upbeat in personality with a true desire to make a difference with the members. This type of staff member employed by the Company is in contrast with the employee of the typical health club. The typical health club hires student interns and struggling dancers or actors to staff their clubs for less money. They cannot be expected to have the science background or experience needed to advise trusting members how to use potentially injury-causing exercise equipment.

The Company will have a proprietary comprehensive internal training program for its staff. These training programs cover all areas of their job description and how management wants them to work with the members of each program. The Company will also provide an incentive plan to the staff for all renewals of membership above a predetermined percentage level of renewals.

A base number of staff are needed to open each center. As each center grows in membership and program offerings, the need develops for more staff, and more staff will be hired to satisfy the facility's requirements.

VI.   MARKET ANALYSIS AND COMPETITION SURVEY

General

The Company will develop its proposed facility in one of the most affluent counties and residential areas in Allendale, New Jersey.

Demographics

The location of the Company's proposed first center will be Allendale, New Jersey. Management performed a demographic survey of the communities within 8 miles of Allendale, New Jersey. Management feels the potential member will travel more than 8 miles for its unique features, but to be conservative management felt it was prudent to use 8 miles for this document. A demographic analysis of Allendale, New Jersey, is attached as Schedule A at the end of this section of this business plan.

Competition Analysis

Management believes several competitive factors influence success in the fitness club business, including convenience, price, customer service, quality of operations, quality of programming, and ability to secure prime real estate at economical rates. We believe that our integrated programming and services focused on enabling our targeted customer base to get results and the price-to-value relationships are very attractive compared to that of our competitors. The combination of an exceptional member experience created through innovative programming, high-quality service and operations, and superior club design will position Triad as one of the few recognized brands within the area. Our offering of ancillary services and products further distinguishes us as a quality brand.

A competition survey of the surrounding area of Allendale, New Jersey, is attached as Schedule B at the end of this section. In this survey, management has picked its unique features that separate the Company from its competition for analysis. This survey reaches out 12 miles from its proposed Allendale location. Having such good access from Route 17, which is a major highway in this area, management feels that its potential members will drive this distance for the Company's unique features.

Adult Physical Fitness

The APFP will attract an exclusive market segment within a 1 – 10-mile radius of its proposed location. The primary target market will be mature, affluent, well-educated, physically deconditioned, overweight men and women 35 years and older who value the importance of personal service, professionally trained staff, and safe, customized, and goal-oriented programs of physical fitness. These potential members frequently have very busy schedules but are serious about getting into and staying in good physical condition so they look better, feel better, and perform better. Today this demographic profile is one of the fastest-growing segments within the United States. The average household income will be $120,000 or more.

Athlete Training Center

The ATC will attract a market segment within a 1 – 30-mile radius of its proposed location. The primary target market will be six market groups: student athletes aged 8–20, recreational athletes, elite, amateur, as well as professional athletes and occupational athletes (people whose jobs require physical strength, speed, and agility) who have a household income of $75,000. In some cases, the athlete will be subsidized by their local school district, town, coach, professional team, or professional agent.

A secondary target market will be off-site Team Camps and Coaches' Clinics delivered by the Director of the ATC. These programs will be on a fee-for-service basis and will further solidify ATC's presence as an "expert" in youth fitness, while broadening its appeal to the community.

Youth Fitness Zone

The YFZ program will attract a market segment within a 1- –20-mile radius of its proposed location. The primary target markets will be (a) children who applied for the ATC and as a result of the assessments it was determined that they do not have the required physical fitness levels to maximize success within that program; therefore this program would be recommended to these children's parents to "get them in shape" for the ATC program, and (b) deconditioned children who are overweight or obese, have multiple health risk factors, and are generally sedentary because of the peer pressure placed on them because of their physical profile or of being less coordinated than their peers. Their ages will range from 5 to 20 whose parents have a household income of $75,000.

VII.   MARKETING AND ADVERTISING PLAN

The Company will retain an experienced advertising agency that has successfully done the advertising for the Physiofitness Centers when they were owned by Mr. Smith and his partners. They will differentiate the Company's services and programs from the "typical health club" market through aggressive, sophisticated targeted advertising and marketing, which will carve out the Company's market niche in this affluent area in New Jersey. The first year's budget for advertising and marketing, which will build brand awareness and turn to member sales, will be $106,100.

We will maintain an ongoing marketing and advertising program aimed at increasing our brand recognition and generating sales prospects. We plan on reaching prospective and existing customers through referrals, direct mail, and print advertising. We also plan on using a billboard on top of the rented location to further advertise our center.

We believe that member referrals and word of mouth are our most effective means of marketing. To foster this cost-effective and efficient source of marketing, we will maintain a number of incentives for existing members to continuously produce new member leads, including a free month's membership or Triad gift cards with monetary credit that can be used to purchase programs, services, or products at our center. Several times a year we also target former members by direct mail.

New Member Programs

As stated earlier, as of December 31, 2002, there were 20,249 health clubs in the United States. Each one of these health clubs markets and advertises differently, with the usual underlying theme of each advertisement and marketing campaign price associated with "sexy"-looking models as members. As a result of the fragmented industry characteristics the Company will clearly differentiate itself from the large-scale fitness companies and the local "Mom and Pop" operators of health clubs. Therefore, in its advertising and marketing programs, the Company must clearly define its breadth and quality of its fitness-related services, overall appearance of facility, and amenities offered, as well as the quality of its staff from a professional and customer service point of view.

The Company's marketing and advertising strategy will be developed to appeal to its primary target market that are mature, affluent, well-educated, physically deconditioned, overweight men and women 35 years and older who value personal service, professionally trained staff, and safe, customized, and goal-oriented programs of physical fitness. These advertisements and marketing programs will be designed and placed with enough repetition to build brand awareness. The marketing and advertising programs will also stress the ease of access to a convenient location, a professionally designed upscale exercise facility, especially designed for very busy people who wish to get in shape and stay in shape in a more time-efficient and controlled manner than the standard health club can provide. It will also stress our policy of limiting membership to a maximum capacity that will assure our members will not be inconvenienced in having to wait to use our exercise equipment or any of our locker room facilities or amenities.

The Company will also advertise and promote its 30-Day Guarantee Program that if the new members for whatever reason do not like the program, they will get a full unconditional refund of the membership fees paid to the Company. The advertising and marketing programs will be designed with a call to action helping the prospective member come to the buying decision that the Company's programs and facilities is the right choice for them to meet their fitness needs and goals for a healthier lifestyle.

A combination of direct mail and print advertising will be used to generate sales leads. The Company's management team and some of its senior staff will be active in community action programs that will generate brand awareness through these public relations efforts.

Programs for Renewals of Existing Members

It must be stated that any advertising and/or marketing that is completed in support of developing a new member base will be seen by the Company's existing members. This advertising and marketing program will in turn reinforce current members' buying decisions. Meeting their expectations will result in satisfied members who will renew their membership.

The management has developed several incentive programs that will aid with existing members' renewal. One example of an incentive program is as follows: if an existing member refers X number of potential members who join the program than at renewal time, the existing member will be given Y number of months free for their referrals or Triad gift cards with monetary credit that can be used to purchase programs, services, or products at our center.

Athlete Training Center

The ATC will focus on two marketing vehicles as its primary source of client leads. They are as follows.

The first marketing vehicle will be newspaper advertising that will help to establish the programs profile in the surrounding communities. The ads will also provide a call to action offering a free in-house seminar — reservation required. Those interested will call in to register for a prescheduled seminar. Registrants will attend the seminar with their child. The seminar will be an introductory orientation to the ATC program, culminating with a call to action to purchase and schedule an athletic assessment.

Those registrants who do not attend or purchase an assessment will be entered into ATC's prospecting "tickler file." They will be mailed a program brochure, and will receive a phone invitation to the next free seminar. Seminars will be regularly scheduled 2 evenings per week.

The second marketing vehicle will be direct marketing to scholastic athletic directors, coaches, and select athletes. The current "Blue Book" (New Jersey State Interscholastic Athletic Association Directory) will be the ideal resource, providing ATC with all contact information for every athletic director and specific sport coaches in the desired target market. ATC will contact athletic directors offering them complimentary Sports Performance Clinics on school grounds. ATC will contact sports coaches to invite them to ATC for Sport-specific Coaches' Clinics. ATC will use the published lists of All-State, All-County, All-League, and Honorable Mentioned high school athletes and target these athletes, inviting them to Scholar-Athlete Clinics at ATC. All of these clinics and seminars are designed to promote and sell the ATC program.

Youth Fitness Zone

YFZ will be actively marketed via three vehicles. The first will be regularly scheduled newspaper advertising in county and community newspapers that will raise the YFZ program profile. The ads will provide a call to action offering a complimentary "first" session. For those who call, they can preregister to reserve a space in a scheduled class of their choice. Registrants who do not attend or enroll upon their visit go into our YFZ prospecting tickler file for ongoing marketing efforts.

The second vehicle will be a promotion directly to principals and teachers of local schools, and community groups (*i.e.*, Rotary Clubs, Lions, Parent Teachers Associations, etc.) via a "Youth Fitness Zone" presentation that will spread the message of the program and motivate parents to register their children in the YFZ program. Attendees will receive a brochure and an "invitation" for their child to attend a complimentary "first session."

Third, a direct marketing campaign will be developed to local pediatricians, providing them with a patient handout for the parents of children needing the YFZ program, which will raise the program's profile with the Doctors and parents.

Demographic Summary: 2002 Estimates
59 STATE RT 17 S: ALLENDALE,NJ 07401
3 Mi Ring (Site located at 41.0428, 74.1156)

Schuyler Companies
06/28/2004

Population		**59,858**	
	In Group Quarters	686	1.1%
Race:	White	55,041	92.0%
	Black	409	0.7%
	American Indian	27	0.0%
	Asian/Pacific Islander	3,427	5.7%
	Other Race	954	
Hispanic Origin		1,772	3.0%
Sex:	Male	29,046	48.5%
	Female	30,812	51.5%
Age:	< 6 Years	5,086	8.5%
	6-11 Years	5,620	9.4%
	12-17 Years	4,680	7.8%
	18-24 Years	3,316	5.5%
	25-34 Years	5,406	9.0%
	35-44 Years	10,637	17.8%
	45-54 Years	9,908	16.6%
	55-64 Years	7,175	12.0%
	65-74 Years	4,312	7.2%
	75-84 Years	2,663	4.4%
	85+ Years	1,055	1.8%
Median Age		40.8	
Households		**21,316**	
	Average Household Size	2.8	
Family Households		16,680	78.3%
	Average Family Size	3.2	
Non-Family Households		4,636	21.7%
	Average Non-Fam HH Size	1.3	
Households by Income			
	$0 - $24,999	1,572	7.4%
	$25,000 - $49,999	2,845	13.3%
	$50,000 - $74,999	3,060	14.4%
	$75,000 - $99,999	2,989	14.0%
	$100,000 +	10,850	50.9%
Average HH Income		$141,652	
Median HH Income		$107,523	
Per Capita Income		$50,960	
Vehicles Available		42,847	
	Average Vehicles/HH	2.0	
Total Housing Units		21,779	
	Owner Occupied	18,943	87.0%
	Renter Occupied	2,373	10.9%
	Vacant	463	2.1%

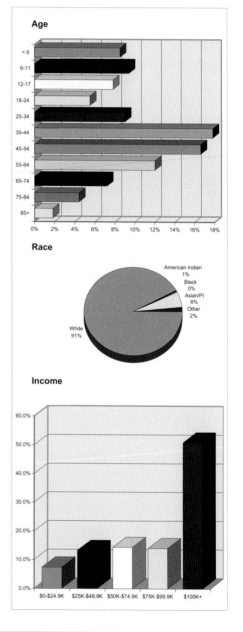

Demographic Summary: 2002 Estimates
59 STATE RT 17 S: ALLENDALE,NJ 07401
6 Mi Ring (Site located at 41.0428, 74.1156)

Schuyler Companies
06/28/2004

Population		**279,787**	
	In Group Quarters	5,258	1.9%
Race:	White	248,326	88.8%
	Black	9,378	3.4%
	American Indian	443	0.2%
	Asian/Pacific Islander	14,585	5.2%
	Other Race	7,055	
Hispanic Origin		13,389	4.8%
Sex:	Male	135,987	48.6%
	Female	143,800	51.4%
Age:	< 6 Years	24,515	8.8%
	6-11 Years	25,317	9.0%
	12-17 Years	23,296	8.3%
	18-24 Years	19,211	6.9%
	25-34 Years	28,651	10.2%
	35-44 Years	46,478	16.6%
	45-54 Years	43,183	15.4%
	55-64 Years	31,249	11.2%
	65-74 Years	20,036	7.2%
	75-84 Years	12,628	4.5%
	85+ Years	5,223	1.9%
Median Age		38.9	
Households		**96,740**	
	Average Household Size	2.8	
Family Households		74,305	76.8%
	Average Family Size	3.3	
Non-Family Households		22,435	23.2%
	Average Non-Fam HH Size	1.4	
Households by Income			
	$0 - $24,999	10,575	10.9%
	$25,000 - $49,999	15,463	16.0%
	$50,000 - $74,999	15,231	15.7%
	$75,000 - $99,999	14,184	14.7%
	$100,000 +	41,287	42.7%
Average HH Income		$117,223	
Median HH Income		$92,520	
Per Capita Income		$40,993	
Vehicles Available		182,069	
	Average Vehicles/HH	1.9	
Total Housing Units		98,778	
	Owner Occupied	78,808	79.8%
	Renter Occupied	17,932	18.2%
	Vacant	2,038	2.1%

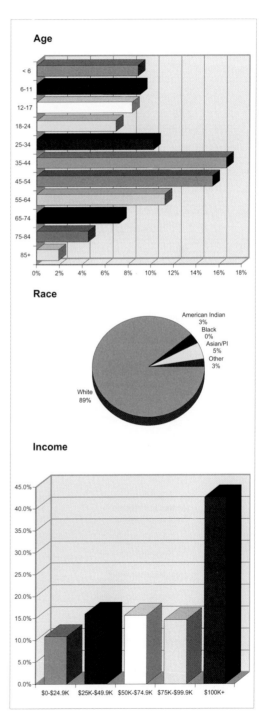

Age

Race

Income

Demographic Summary: 2002 Estimates
59 STATE RT 17 S: ALLENDALE,NJ 07401
9 Mi Ring (Site located at 41.0428, 74.1156)

Schuyler Companies
06/28/2004

Population		**635,595**	
	In Group Quarters	14,128	2.2%
Race:	White	502,259	79.0%
	Black	58,856	9.3%
	American Indian	1,218	0.2%
	Asian/Pacific Islander	37,639	5.9%
	Other Race	35,623	
Hispanic Origin		58,273	9.2%
Sex:	Male	306,666	48.2%
	Female	328,929	51.8%
Age:	< 6 Years	55,195	8.7%
	6-11 Years	57,484	9.0%
	12-17 Years	54,065	8.5%
	18-24 Years	48,506	7.6%
	25-34 Years	69,575	10.9%
	35-44 Years	101,968	16.0%
	45-54 Years	94,435	14.9%
	55-64 Years	68,460	10.8%
	65-74 Years	44,825	7.1%
	75-84 Years	29,140	4.6%
	85+ Years	11,942	1.9%
Median Age		38.0	
Households		**214,297**	
	Average Household Size	2.9	
Family Households		165,083	77.0%
	Average Family Size	3.3	
Non-Family Households		49,214	23.0%
	Average Non-Fam HH Size	1.5	
Households by Income			
	$0 - $24,999	30,794	14.4%
	$25,000 - $49,999	38,269	17.9%
	$50,000 - $74,999	36,643	17.1%
	$75,000 - $99,999	30,978	14.5%
	$100,000 +	77,611	36.2%
Average HH Income		$100,982	
Median HH Income		$81,728	
Per Capita Income		$34,515	
Vehicles Available		387,067	
	Average Vehicles/HH	1.8	
Total Housing Units		219,606	
	Owner Occupied	161,508	73.5%
	Renter Occupied	52,789	24.0%
	Vacant	5,309	2.4%

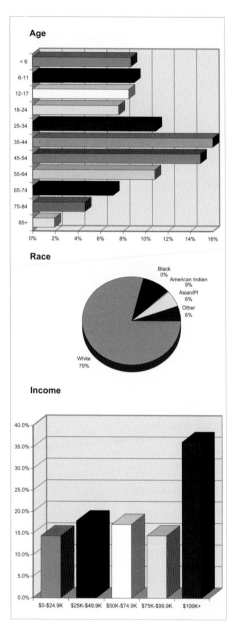

Demographic Summary: 2002 Estimates
59 STATE RT 17 S: ALLENDALE,NJ 07401
12 Mi Ring (Site located at 41.0428, 74.1156)

Population	**1,193,290**	
In Group Quarters	25,252	2.1%
Race: White	891,835	74.7%
Black	113,616	9.5%
American Indian	2,909	0.2%
Asian/Pacific Islander	76,359	6.4%
Other Race	108,571	
Hispanic Origin	**171,686**	14.4%
Sex: Male	577,107	48.4%
Female	616,183	51.6%
Age: < 6 Years	98,672	8.3%
6-11 Years	102,360	8.6%
12-17 Years	98,045	8.2%
18-24 Years	95,796	8.0%
25-34 Years	143,370	12.0%
35-44 Years	192,872	16.2%
45-54 Years	176,145	14.8%
55-64 Years	125,100	10.5%
65-74 Years	82,133	6.9%
75-84 Years	55,906	4.7%
85+ Years	22,891	1.9%
Median Age	**38.0**	
Households	**410,925**	
Average Household Size	2.8	
Family Households	**304,935**	74.2%
Average Family Size	3.3	
Non-Family Households	**105,990**	25.8%
Average Non-Fam HH Size	1.5	
Households by Income		
$0 - $24,999	66,574	16.2%
$25,000 - $49,999	83,780	20.4%
$50,000 - $74,999	75,172	18.3%
$75,000 - $99,999	59,100	14.4%
$100,000 +	126,286	30.7%
Average HH Income	**$90,000**	
Median HH Income	**$73,697**	
Per Capita Income	**$31,439**	
Vehicles Available	**707,016**	
Average Vehicles/HH	1.7	
Total Housing Units	**422,381**	
Owner Occupied	281,474	66.6%
Renter Occupied	129,451	30.6%
Vacant	11,456	2.7%

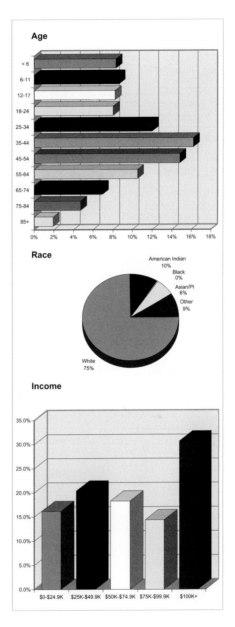

Age

Race

Income

Demographic Summary: 2002 Estimates
59 STATE RT 17 S: ALLENDALE,NJ 07401
15 Mi Ring (Site located at 41.0428, 74.1156)

Schuyler Companies
06/28/2004

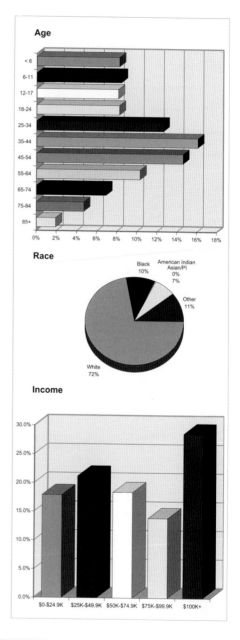

Population	**1,810,377**	
In Group Quarters	36,178	2.0%
Race: White	1,307,200	72.2%
Black	177,993	9.8%
American Indian	4,934	0.3%
Asian/Pacific Islander	122,876	6.8%
Other Race	197,374	
Hispanic Origin	309,170	17.1%
Sex: Male	874,127	48.3%
Female	936,250	51.7%
Age: < 6 Years	148,759	8.2%
6-11 Years	152,627	8.4%
12-17 Years	146,409	8.1%
18-24 Years	147,660	8.2%
25-34 Years	228,053	12.6%
35-44 Years	291,594	16.1%
45-54 Years	263,865	14.6%
55-64 Years	186,560	10.3%
65-74 Years	124,249	6.9%
75-84 Years	85,711	4.7%
85+ Years	34,890	1.9%
Median Age	37.8	
Households	**634,199**	
Average Household Size	2.8	
Family Households	458,532	72.3%
Average Family Size	3.3	
Non-Family Households	175,667	27.7%
Average Non-Fam HH Size	1.5	
Households by Income		
$0 - $24,999	113,736	17.9%
$25,000 - $49,999	134,483	21.2%
$50,000 - $74,999	116,690	18.4%
$75,000 - $99,999	88,184	13.9%
$100,000 +	181,081	28.6%
Average HH Income	$86,146	
Median HH Income	$70,020	
Per Capita Income	$30,623	
Vehicles Available	1,034,179	
Average Vehicles/HH	1.6	
Total Housing Units	653,425	
Owner Occupied	404,469	61.9%
Renter Occupied	229,730	35.2%
Vacant	19,226	2.9%

Scan/US, Inc. 310.820.1581   Source: Scan/US 2002 Estimates   www.scanus.com

VIII. SCHEDULE B — COMPETITIVE SURVEY OF ALLENDALE, NEW JERSEY, AND SURROUNDING AREAS

Name of Club	Distance from 59 Route 17 South Allendale, NJ	Address	Adult Fitness Program Enrollment Fee	Adult Fitness Program Annual Fee Pd Upfront	Adult Fitness Program Monthly Fee	Discount to Pay Upfront	Ongoing Professionally Supervised Exercise Programming	Degreed Exercise Physiology Staff	Adult Member Attendance Follow-up Program	Children's Training and or Remedial Programs	Amount Charged for Children's Training & Conditioning Programming	Assessment for Children's Training & Conditioning Programming
Triad Fitness	**0 mi.**	**59 Route 17 South, Allendale, NJ**	**$99**	**$960**	**$80**	**0.00%**	**Yes**	**Yes**	**Yes**	**Yes**	**$30 for 12 Sessions and $28.95 for 24 Sessions**	**$95**
Odyssey Health and Fitness	1.5mi.	168 Franklin Turnpike, Waldwick	$99	$600	$55 Per Month or $660/Yr.	10.00%	No	No	No	No	N/A	N/A
NY Sports Club	2.7mi.	1150 Highway 17, Ramsey	$99	N/A	$75 Per Month or $900/Yr.	N/A	No	No	No	No	N/A	N/A
FlexPlex Health & Fitness	3.3mi.	150 Triangle 17 Plaza, Ramsey	$100	N/A	$59 Per Month or $708/Yr.	0.00%	No	No	No	No	N/A	N/A
The Gym	4.4mi.	2 Chestnut Ridge Road, Montvale	$99	N/A	$80 Per Month or $960/Yr.	0.00%	No	No	No	No	N/A	N/A
NY Sports Club	5.1mi.	129 South Broad St. Ridgewood	$99	N/A	$84 Per Month or $900/Yr.	N/A	No	No	No	No	N/A	N/A
World's Gym	7.4mi.	600 Winters Ave. Paramus	$99	$699	$59 Pd Monthly or $708/Yr	1.27%	No	No	No	No	N/A	N/A
Westwood Health and Fitness	7.9mi.	346 Kinderkamack Rd. Westwood	N/A	$720	$65 Pd Monthly or $780/Yr	7.69%	No	No	No	No	N/A	N/A
Gold's Gym	7.9mi.	49 East Midland Ave. Paramus	N/A	$599	$69 Pd Monthly or $828/Yr	27.65%	No	No	No	No	N/A	N/A
NY Sports Club (A)	8.1mi.	Jefferson Ave. Westwood	$99	N/A	$75 Per Month or $900/Yr	N/A	No	No	No	Yes Swim Lessons Only	N/A	N/A
Health Spa 2	11.0mi	Route 4 and Forrest Ave. Paramus	$99	$699	$59 Per Month or $708/Yr	1.27%	No	No	No	No	N/A	N/A
Body Designs	11.4mi.	224 Route 4, Paramus	$99	$720	$70 Pd Monthly or $840/Yr	14.28%	No	No	No	No	N/A	N/A
Parisi's	11.8mi.	2-22 Banta Place, Fairlawn	$99	$714	$59.50 Per Month or 714/Yr	0.00%	No	No	Yes	Yes - Sports Training Program No - Remedial Program	$32.92 for 12 Sessions and $31.46 for 24 Sessions	$95

Notes

Competition Survey only includes Health Clubs with comparable facilities & programs to those proposed by The Company

(A) To be opened on or before April 2004

Competition survey of Allendale, New Jersey, and surrounding areas.

IX. USE OF FUNDS: ABC FITNESS CAPITAL AND STARTUP BUDGET

Start Up Items	Month 1	Month 2	Month 3	Month 4	Month 5	Month 6	Sub-Totals of Start Up Items	1st FY: Ongoing use of Working Capital	Total Capital Needed
Construction Costs & Construction Contingency	$ 229,688	$ 229,688	$ 229,688	$ 229,688	$ 229,688	$ 229,688	$ 1,378,125		$ 1,378,125
Architects Fee	$ 21,875	$ 21,875	$ 21,875	$ 21,875	$ 21,875	$ 21,875	$ 131,250		$ 131,250
Engineers Fee	$ 9,844	$ 9,844	$ 9,844			$ 9,844	$ 39,375		$ 39,375
Signage - Internal & External				$ 3,000	$ 12,000		$ 15,000		$ 15,000
Misc Consultants- Expediter, Graphics, etc.	$ 2,188	$ 2,188	$ 2,188				$ 6,563		$ 6,563
Exercise & Related Equipment: 1st & Last Month Deposit on Lease		$ 21,504					$ 21,504		$ 21,504
Start Up Costs - Non Capital	$ 55,385	$ 55,385	$ 55,385	$ 55,385	$ 55,385	$ 55,385	$ 332,311		$ 332,311
Ongoing use of Working Capital								$ 200,000	$ 200,000
Totals	$ 318,979	$ 340,483	$ 321,979	$ 306,948	$ 318,948	$ 316,791	$ 1,924,128	$ 200,000	$ 2,124,128

Start-up cash flow.

Total Square Feet		17,500	
Construction Costs per Sq FT	$ 75.00		
Capital Costs			
Construction & Related Costs	Budget	Total within each Area	
Construction Costs	$ 1,312,500		
Construction Contingency: 5% of Cons't Costs	$ 65,625		
Architects Fee: 10% of Cons't Costs	$ 131,250		
Engineers Fee: 3% of Cons't Costs	$ 39,375		
Signage - Internal & External	$ 15,000		
Misc Consultants- Expediter, Graphics, etc.: 0.5% of Cons't Costs	$ 6,563		
Sub-Total Construction & Related Costs		$ 1,570,313	$ 104,688
15 Yrs Amortization			$ 10,000 — 10 Yrs Professional Fees
			$ 114,688 — 15 Yr Amortization
Exercise & Related Equipment	Items to be Leased		
Accessories	$ 9,446		
Broadcast Vision	$ 52,004		
Cardiovascular Equipment	$ 227,559		
Computer & Office Hardware	$ 35,739		
Computer Software	$ 15,960		
Free Weights and Plate Loaded Equipment	$ 35,216		
Group Classroom Equipment	$ 28,187		
Laundry Room and Storage Equipment	$ 19,372		
Selectorized Strength Equipment	$ 108,828		
Athlete Training Center	$ 25,477		
Testing Equipment	$ 3,198		
Total Exercise & Related Equipment	$ 560,985		
1st & Last Month Deposit on Lease		$ 21,504	
7 Yr Depreciation			$ 80,141 — 7 Yr Depreciation
Start Up Costs - Non Capital	Budget		
Locker Amenities and Hygienic Supplies	$ 16,791		
Member Towels	$ 13,488		
Staff Uniforms	$ 2,200		
Office supplies	$ 10,000		
Salaries			
Smith - 6 months	$ 37,500		
Milkin - 6 months	$ 37,500		
Pirelli - 4 months	$ 25,000		
2 F/T Ex Phys - 1 Month	$ 6,251		
2 F/T Admin Assist for Adult & STA - 1 Month	$ 4,840		
2 F/T LRA - 1 Month	$ 3,987		
4 P/T Receptionists for Mon-Sun - 2 Weeks	$ 1,328		
2 P/T LRA for Sat & Sun - 2 Weeks	$ 440		
2 P/T Ex Phys for Sat & Sun - 2 Weeks	$ 616		
Sub-Total Salaries		$ 117,461	
Payroll Taxes 10%	$ 11,746		
Advertising, Marketing & Promotion	$ 45,000		
Professional Fees	$ 50,000		
Rent Security Deposit	$ 65,625		
Sub-Total Non Capital Start Up Costs		$ 332,311	
Working Capital			
1st Year Requirements	$ 200,000	$ 200,000	
Total Capital Funds Needed		$ 2,124,128	

Summary.

Item - Accessory				
Manufacterer	**Model #**	**Qty**	**Unit Cost**	**Cost**
Magazine racks and covers	TBD	4	$ 75	$ 300
Sub-Total				**$ 300**
Umbra				
Verra Photo Frame	316364 (656 Walnut)	1	$ 8	$ 8
Bullet Board	035515 (15"x 21" Nickel)	4	$ 15	$ 60
Flex Mirror	022430 (410 Nickel)	6	$ 25	$ 150
Single Wall Hook	022401 (410 Nickel)	48	$ 4	$ 168
Wall Shelf	022415 (410 Nickel)	3	$ 20	$ 60
Spin Wall Clock	118335 (008 Aluminum - 9.5" dia)	9	$ 8	$ 68
Station Wall Clock	118675 (008 Aluminum - 14.5" dia)	10	$ 30	$ 300
Beam Desk Clock	114080 (008 Aluminum)	4	$ 10	$ 40
Stream Pivot Wall Mirror	358540 (410 Nickel)	2	$ 25	$ 50
Step Can	084803 (.560 Silver)	3	$ 10	$ 30
Replacement Cartridge (preferred 250)		4	$ 95	$ 380
Sub-Total				**$ 1,313**
American Hotel Registry				
Shoe Shine - Standing Electric	55J-795	2	$ 90	$ 180
Shoe Shine - Black Replacement Bonnet	55J-Black	2	$ 16	$ 32
Shoe Shine - Red Replacement Bonnett	55J-Red	2	$ 16	$ 32
Q-tip holder	A58-1227	6	$ 11	$ 66
Curling Iron		4	$ 25	$ 100
Shoe Horns - dozen (p.665)	MZC-LB (3 in 1 shoe horn)	12	$ 6	$ 66
Shoe Horns - dozen (p.665)	X6H-M7ESA (3 gross)	1	$ 80	$ 80
Tiered Clothing Hanger - retail		2	$ 150	$ 300
Wooden Hangers (Walnut/Mohogany)	CL7K-70-DBW	2	$ 100	$ 200
Wooden Hangers (Walnut/Mohogany)	CL7K-70-WNS	2	$ 110	$ 220
Personal Steamer (p.1759)	MZL-ESTEAM	1	$ 80	$ 80
Wall Mount Corkboards	P4C-AK-44	1	$ 74	$ 74
Wall Mount Corkboards	P4C-1330-1	1	$ 45	$ 45
Designer Waste Receptacles	FGM-F2035	2	$ 265	$ 530
Structural Foam - Cubic Yard Tilt Truck	S5R-1011	1	$ 468	$ 468
Hinged Dome Lid for Tilt Truck	S5R-1028	1	$ 133	$ 133
Hair Dryers	Andis- 1600	16	$ 55	$ 880
Compact Discs-		100	$ 18	$ 1,800
AED	American Red Cross	1	$ 3,000	$ 3,000
Sub-Total				**$ 8,286**
Sub-Total				**$ 8,286**
NJ Sales Tax @ 6%				**$ 497**
Freight @ 8%				**$ 663**
Total				**$ 9,446**

Accessories.

Item - Broadcast Vision		Quantity	Unit	Cost
Broadcast Vision	PFC Units- monitor	34	$ 935	$ 31,790
Broadcast Vision	PFC Units- stand	34	$ 102	$ 3,468
Setup Remote		1	$ 15	$ 15
Installation				$ 6,000
Sub-Total				**$ 41,273**
NJ Sales Tax @ 6%				**$ 2,476**
Freight @ 8%				**$ 3,302**
Instillation @ 10%				**$ 4,127**
Contingency @ 2%				**$ 825**
Total				**$ 52,004**

Broadcast vision.

Item - Cardiovascular Training Equipment	Qty	Unit Cost	Cost	
Treadmills & Like				
Precor C956 Treadmill with HHHR- 220 volts	6	$ 4,695	$ 28,170	
TrueTreadmill- 110 volts	6	$ 4,600	$ 27,600	
Precor EFX 546	6	$ 3,895	$ 23,370	
Precor EFX 556 Total Body	6	$ 3,895	$ 23,370	
Sub-Total				$ 102,510
Bikes				
Precor Recumbent- black frame	8	$ 2,200	**$ 17,600**	
Precor Upright- black frame	8	$ 2,050	**$ 16,400**	
Cybex Tectrix Climbmax 800	8	$ 2,400	**$ 19,200**	
Sub-Total				$ 53,200
StairMasters				
StepMill	1	$ 3,995	$ 3,995	
Regular StairMasters	5	$ 2,500	$ 12,500	
Sub-Total				$ 16,495
Rowing Units				
Concept II Rower	4	$ 950	$ 3,800	
Sub-Total				$ 3,800
Miscel CV Exercise Equip				
Precor Stretch Trainer	1	$ 595	$ 595	
Versa Climber	2	$ 2,900	$ 5,800	
Cycle Plus	2	$ 4,050	$ 8,100	
UBE	1	$ 3,995	$ 3,995	
Sub-Total				$ 18,490
Sub-Total of All Cardiovascular Equip				$ 194,495
NJ Sales Tax @ 6%				$ 11,670
Freight & Installation @ 9%				$ 17,505
Contingency @ 2%				$ 3,890
Total				$ 227,559

Cardiovascular equipment.

Item - Computers & Office Hardware	Unit Cost	Quantity	Cost
Compaq Desktop Computers **(A)**	1,000	8	$ 8,000
HP 4050TN Networked Laser Printer	1,600	1	$ 1,600
17" Flat Panel	700	8	$ 5,600
HP Color Laserjet 4550N	2,250	1	$ 2,250
Compaq Proliant Server	3,500	1	$ 3,500
Tape backup system	900	1	$ 900
Copier, Fax, Scanner & Printer - 1 Unit from Xerox	4,000	1	$ 4,000
Misc.			$ 3,000
Installation			$ 2,500
Sub-Total			**$ 31,350**
NJ Sales Tax @ 6%			**$ 1,881**
Freight & Installation @ 8%			**$ 2,508**
Total			**$ 35,739**
(A) Checkin Adult, Checkin Children, 3-Managers Office, 2 Fitness Area, 1-Member Program Area			

Computers and office hardware.

Item - Computer Software	Unit Cost	Quantity	Cost
Software licenses- Club Management System			$ 10,000
Card Integrators	0.50	2,000	$ 1,000
Office Licenses			$ 3,000
Sub-Total			**$ 14,000**
NJ Sales Tax @ 6%			**$ 840**
Freight & Installation @ 8%			**$ 1,120**
Total			**$ 15,960**

Computer software.

Item - Free Weight Equipment	Unit	Model #	Qty	Unit	Cost	
Plate loaded Manufacturer						
Cybex	Smith Machine	5,341	2	$2,050	$4,100	
Cybex	Power Rack	5,420	2	$1,050	$2,100	
Cybex	Olympic Bench Press	5,350	1	$600	$600	
Cybex	Olympic Incline Bench Press	5,370	1	$690	$690	
Cybex	Olympic Adjustable Bench Decline to Incline		2	$750	$1,500	
Cybex	Weight Tree w/barbell holder	5,490	4	$265	$1,060	
Cybex	Preacher Curl	5,460	1	$435	$435	
Sub-Total						$10,485
Free Weights Manufacturer						
Magnum	2 tier- 15 pr Dumbbell Rack	M42	4	$215	**$860**	
CAP Rubber Hex	Dumbbells 3,5,8,10,12,15,20,25,…110	CAP	4		**$5,500**	
Hampton	8pr Dumbbell rack		3	$210	**$630**	
Cybex	Adjustable Benches- flat -90degrees	5,345	8	$500	**$4,000**	
Cybex	Upright Bench	5,520	1	$265	**$265**	
Power Sys.	Step-Up Box		1	$150	**$150**	
Iron Grip	45 pound plates		30	$56	**$1,688**	
Iron Grip	35 pound plates		4	$44	**$175**	
Iron Grip	25 pound plates		16	$31	**$500**	
Iron Grip	10 pound plates		16	$13	**$200**	
Iron Grip	5 pound plates		16	$6	**$100**	
Iron Grip	2.5 pound plates		4	$3	**$13**	
Cybex	45 Degree back extension	5,411	1	$535	**$535**	
Sub-Total						$14,615
Power Systems						
	Foot air pump	80,095	2	$20	$40	
	Ball stackers	81,010	1	$40	$40	
	Wobble and rocker boards	80,390	1	$230	$230	
	Power Med. Balls 4,6,8,10,12	25,010	2	$16	$32	
		25,020	2	$20	$40	
		25,030	2	$30	$60	
		25,040	2	$40	$80	
		25,050	2	$50	$100	
	Medicine ball rebounder	21,060	1	$450	$450	
	Medicine ball Double Tree	6719P	1	$160	$160	
	Power vest	1,310	1	$90	$90	
	Step up box	40,210	1	$169	$169	
	Plastic Quicklee collars	50,420	10	$20	$200	
	Muscle clamps	50,450	10	$30	$300	
	Pro style 36in. Lat bar	60,805	1	$38	$38	
	Revolving curl bar	60,810	1	$33	$33	
	24" Pro style lat bar	60,820	1	$38	$38	
	34" Pro Style lat bar	60,825	1	$40	$40	
	Pro tricep press down	60,840	2	$20	$40	
	Pro revolving press down bar	60,835	1	$30	$30	
	Pro revolving multi exercise bar	60,845	1	$40	$40	
	Pro seated low row bar	60,850	2	$20	$40	
	Pro delux single grip handles	60,855	2	$25	$50	
	Pro Tricep rope	50,740	1	$25	$25	
	Super Tricep rope	50,745	1	$40	$40	
	Power rope	35,502	1	$26	$26	
	Power rope	35,503	1	$30	$30	
	6" Nylon Belt med	65,080	1	$25	$25	
	6" Nylon Belt large	65,080	1	$25	$25	
	6" Nylon Belt xl	65,080	1	$25	$25	
	Shoulder horn-m to l	67,000	1	$60	$60	
	Pro Abdominator	67,112	1	$50	$50	
	Hand Wraps	92,175	12	$4	$47	
Sub-Total						$2,693
Gym Source	Hausman cuff weights - 1-10lbs.	5,580 (1-10)	1	$400	$400	
	Hausman cuff weight rack	5,565	1	$300	$300	
	Airex mats- Coronella		6	$80	$480	
	ez curl bar		2	$85	$170	
	barbell neck roll pads		3	$12	$36	
	35 pound olympic bar (chrome)		1	$130	$130	
	45 pound olympic bar (Chrome)		6	$175	$1,050	
Sub-Total						$2,566
Sub-Total						$30,359
NJ Sales Tax @ 6%						$1,822
Freight & Installation @ 8%						$2,429
Contingency @ 2%						$607
Total						$35,216

Free weights.

Item - Group Class Equipment	Item	Model #	Qty	Unit cost	Cost	
Gym Source						
Star Trac	Spinning bike	V Bike	16	$675	$10,800	
King	Body Bar rack		1	$385	$385	
Everlast	Training Gloves	4306	12	$29	$348	
Everlast	Target Mitts	4315	4	$48	$192	
Everlast	Boxing Gloves	2078	4	$40	$160	
Nevertear DE	Mobile Heavy Bags		4	$140	$560	
Sub-Total						$12,445
Spri						
Step Company	The Step	OCS	24	$49	$1,176	
Step Company	Risers (pairs)	OCSR	48	$10	$480	
Neoprene dumbells- pairs						
2lb		db-2	16	$8	$128	
4lb		db-4	16	$11	$176	
6lb		db-6	12	$15	$180	
8lb		db-8	12	$18	$216	
10lb		db-10	12	$21	$252	
Premium weight rack		DBR-D	1	$250	$250	
Spri Hugger Mugger		FB-P	14	$13	$181	
Spri blanket		WB	10	$20	$200	
Sub-Total						$3,239
Fitness Wholesale						
Fitness Step mats		FMSTPDL	24	$10	$228	
Theraband balls		FBS 55	6	$14	$84	
		FBS 65	6	$18	$108	
Body Bars		Bar 9	8	$24	$192	
		Bar 12	8	$27	$216	
		Bar 15	8	$30	$240	
		Bar 18	7	$33	$231	
		Bar 22D	7	$49	$343	
		Bar 24D	2	$49	$99	
Tubing w/ Tube gaurds		TG2LT	15	$5	$68	
		TG2MD	12	$6	$69	
		TG2HV	12	$6	$72	
Ultra Mats		TAPUM	1	$30	$30	
Vinyl Speed Ropes		EXJ08	12	$2	$22	
		EXJ09	12	$2	$23	
		EXJ10	12	$2	$24	
Pro Stretch		PROST	2	$19	$38	
Sub-Total						$2,086
Metro	Studio Aerobic Shelves	86P	8	$ 23	$ 184	
Metro		A3072NC	8	$ 139	$ 1,112	
Metro		L72N-IC	8	$ 18	$ 144	
Metro		HK25C	15	$ 3	$ 45	
Metro	Training Floor Carts	MW703	2	$ 270	$ 540	
Metro	Reception	74P	4	$ 19	$ 76	
Metro		A2448NC	2	$ 78	$ 156	
Metro		1AT4824NC	1	$ 29	$ 29	
Metro	Staff Closet	74P	8	$ 19	$ 152	
Metro		A1836NC	6	$ 54	$ 324	
Metro		AT3618NC	1	$ 27	$ 27	
Metro	Spa Closet	74P	4	$ 19	$ 76	
Metro		A1848NC	4	$ 63	$ 252	
Metro		1836NC wall mount	2	$ 50	$ 100	
Metro		SW33C wall count	1	$ 194	$ 194	
Metro	Locker Room	86P	8	$ 23	$ 184	
Metro		A2148NC	8	$ 71	$ 568	
Metro		SF45N3C	1	$ 54	$ 54	
Metro	Towel Cart	AST55DC	1	$ 803	$ 803	
Sub-Total						$ 5,020
Miscl Items						
Maximum Performance Al ropes			20	$ 10	$ 200	
CD's					$ 314	
Dynamix CD's					$ 212	
Pilates equipment					$ 559	
Reebok Core board					$ 225	
Sub-Total						$ 1,510
Sub-Total						$ 24,299
NJ Sales Tax @ 6%						$1,458
Freight & Installation @ 8%						$1,944
Contingency @ 2%						$486
Total						$28,187

Group classroom equipment.

Item - Laundry & Storage		Quantity	Unit Cost		Cost	
Description		Quantity	Unit Cost		Cost	
Metro						
48X24X84 Shelving w/board	44605T61	3	$	129	$	1,100
Staff Fridge					$	200
Microwave					$	225
reception fridge					$	1,000
Heavy Duty Tuflite Polyethylene Laundry trucks	p/n W6S - 3910X1	1			$	175
50lb Wascomat Washer*		2	$	3,000	$	6,000
75lb Wascomat Dryer*		2	$	4,000	$	8,000
Sub-Total					**$ 16,700**	
NJ Sales Tax @ 6%					**$ 1,002**	
Freight & Installation @ 10%					**$ 1,670**	
Total					**$ 19,372**	

Laundry and storage.

Item - Selectorized Strength Training						
Manufacturer	**Unit**	model #	Qty	Unit Cost	Cost	
Cybex Eagle	Seated Leg Curl w/ total RDL		2	$2,660	$5,320	
Cybex Eagle	Leg Extension w/total RDL		2	$2,660	$5,320	
Cybex Eagle	Leg Curl w/total RDL		2	$2,600	$5,200	
Cybex Eagle	Seated Leg Press		2	$3,995	$7,990	
Cybex Eagle	Adductor		2	$2,395	$4,790	
Cybex Eagle	Abductor		2	$2,395	$4,790	
Cybex Eagle	Lat Pulldown		2	$1,725	$1,725	
Cybex Eagle	Seated Row		2	$2,660	$5,320	
Cybex Eagle	Chest Press		2	$2,660	$5,320	
Cybex Eagle	Shoulder Press		2	$2,495	$4,990	
Nautilus	Chin Dip Assist		2	$2,150	$4,300	
Cybex Eagle	Upper Back		2	$2,395	$4,790	
Cybex Eagle	Arm Extension		2	$2,395	$4,790	
Cybex Eagle	Arm Curl		2	$2,395	$4,790	
Cybex Eagle	Ab Crunch		2	$2,395	$4,790	
Cybex Eagle	Lower back		2	$2,395	$4,790	
Free Motion	Cable Crossover with all attachments	6006	2	$3,750	$7,500	
Free Motion	Squat	6001	2	$3,250	$6,500	
Sub-Total					$93,015	
NJ Sales Tax @ 6%					$ 5,581	
Freight & Installation @ 9%					$ 8,371	
Contingency @ 2%					$ 1,860	
Total					$ 108,828	

Selectorized strength.

Items for Sports Training Academy	Unit Cost	
Strength / Power Training Equipment		
Power Rack	$ 550	
Adjustable bench (flat to decline)	$ 750	
Olympic bar	$ 110	
Olympic plates	$ 1,073	
Olympic racks (4) + 2 bar/plate racks	$ 640	
Olympic lifting platform	$ 1,255	
Ivanko rubberized Olympic plates and racks	$ 1,200	
olympic Bar & Training Plates (2)	$ 150	
Powerblocks #45Lb (4)	$ 876	
Reverse-hyper	$ 1,500	
Power Runner	$ 2,500	
Power sled (4 @ $180)	$ 720	
Chains	$ 200	
Bands	$ 200	
Glute/Ham bench	$ 800	
Deadlift bar (2)	$ 320	
Cable Crossover with all attachments		
Squat		
Sub-Total		$ 12,844
Agility-related equipment		
ABC - Agility ladders (4)	$ 360	
Agility cones (24 @ $6)	$ 144	
Mini-hurdles (24 @ $8)	$ 192	
Juke - Breakaway straps (6 @ 15)	$ 90	
Power plyo hurdles (12 @ $27.95)	$ 335	
Plyo Boxes (2ea. 6", 12", 18")	$ 840	
Sub-Total		$ 1,961
Testing Equipment		
Functional testing/training grid	$ 229	
Vertec (vertical jump appraiser)	$ 495	
Muscle Lab Power system	$ 995	
Goniometer	$ 22	
Spring-loaded tape measure	$ 23	
Lange skin-fold caliper	$ 240	
Medical scale	$ 295	
Accusplit stopwatches (4 @ $20)	$ 80	
Speedtrap II Timing system (complete)	$ 1,974	
Sub-Total		$ 4,353
Functional Training equipment		
Power wheel	$ 40	
Power Systems med balls 2ea. (2, 4, 6, 8, 10Lbs)	$ 172	
Med ball double tree	$ 110	
Sidestep (12 @ $40)	$ 480	
JC All-purpose exercise bands (6@25)	$ 150	
JC Quad bands (4@30)	$ 120	
UltraSlide Board	$ 600	
Airex pads (6 @$50)	$ 300	
Wobble/Rocker boards w/stand	$ 220	
Stability Ball Plus (6 ea 55cm & 65cm)	$ 360	
Ball racks (2)	$ 230	
Ball pump	$ 23	
Sub-Total		$ 2,805
Sub-Total		$ 21,963
NJ Sales Tax @ 6%		$ 1,318
Freight & Installation @ 8%		$ 1,757
Contingency @ 2%		439
Total		$ 25,477

Athlete training center.

Item - Testing Equipment		Quantity	Unit		Cost	
Manufacturer						
Lange	Skinfold Caliper	2	$	250	$	500
	Blood Pressure Stand - Mercury	4	$	200	$	800
	1 large bp cuff	4	$	50	$	200
	1small bp cuff	4	$	45	$	180
Detecto	medical scale	3	$	299	$	897
	Stethescopes	6	$	30	$	180
Sub-Total					$	2,757
NJ Sales Tax @ 6%						$165
Freight & Installation @ 8%						$221
Contingency @ 2%						$55
Total					$	3,198

Testing equipment.

Item - Locker Amenities & Supplies	Model #	Quantity	Unit Cost	Cost	
Men's and Women's Shower Dispensers					
Bottles and Labels					
body soap- 32oz bottle		40	$ 27	$ 1,080	
shampoo -32 oz bottle		40	$ 27	$ 1,080	
conditioner- 32oz bottle		40	$ 27	$ 1,080	
3 bottle acrylic dispenser for 32 oz.		40	$ 27	$ 1,078	
Sub-Total					$ 4,318
Men's and Women's Counter Top Bottles					
and Labels					
antimicrobial soap- 32oz bottles		15	$ 1	$ 15	
mouthwash- 32oz bottles		15	$ 1	$ 15	
lotion- 32 oz bottles		15	$ 1	$ 15	
3 bottle acrylic dispenser for 32 oz.		15	$ 27	$ 404	
Sub-Total					$ 449
Consumables for Start Up					
Moisturizing Body Bath Gallons (white soap only)		28	$ 13	$ 375	
Shampoo (1 case of 4 gallons)		4	$ 11	$ 45	
Shampoo (one 30 gallon drum)		2	$ 282	$ 564	
Conditioner (1 case of 4 gallons)		4	$ 11	$ 45	
Conditioner (one 30 gallon drum)		2	$ 282	$ 564	
Antimicrobial Soap (1 case of 4 gallons)		1	$ 12	$ 12	
Antimicrobial Soap (one 30 gallon drum)		2	$ 289	$ 578	
Drum Pump (stainless steal and plastic)		3	$ 48	$ 143	
Mouthwash		18	$ 11	$ 204	
Moisturizing Lotion		18	$ 12	$ 215	
Antiperspirant		8	$ 20	$ 158	
Hairspray		8	$ 17	$ 133	
Men's Razors/ Gillette Custom Plus Pivot				$ -	
Mouthwash cups (1,000 per)		3	$ 20	$ 60	
Mouthwash cups dispenser		3	$ 31	$ 93	
Q Tips Cotton Swabs (170 per)		24	$ 2	$ 39	
Combs (144 per)		1	$ 19	$ 19	
Brushes (#87 Navy, 12 per case, Navy Blue)		6	$ 20	$ 119	
Barbaside containers		12	$ 11	$ 136	
Barbaside liquid		30	$ 13	$ 383	
Smack A Germ (lemon)	N/A	1	$ 36	$ 36	
Latex Gloves Medium	SFS330	2	$ 13	$ 26	
Latex Gloves Large	SFS440	2	$ 13	$ 26	
Cotton Band Mop Head	LBI524C	1	$ 6	$ 6	
Industrial Dust Head	LBI1036	1	$ 10	$ 10	
Dust Mop Frame	LBI1236	1	$ 5	$ 5	
Dust Mop Handle	LBI1490	1	$ 9	$ 9	
Mop Bucket & Wringer	RCP7577YEL	1	$ 80	$ 80	
Wooden Mop Handle	RCPH116	2	$ 9	$ 19	
Lobby Dust Pan	RCP2531	1	$ 14	$ 14	
Lambs wool Extension Duster	DUSL3060	2	$ 9	$ 18	
Maid's Broom	BRM920Y	1	$ 5	$ 5	
Furniture Dusting	DYA32420	1	$ 35	$ 35	
Trigger Spray	LAG7210-8	3	$ 1	$ 4	
24oz. Spray Bottle	LAG 24	3	$ 1	$ 2	
Pullman-Holt Wet/Dry Vacuum	PULEVAC11-15	1	$ 515	$ 515	
Item - Locker Amenities & Supplies	Model #	Quantity	Unit Cost	Cost	
Ajax Multi- Surface Cleaner	SPC04199	1	$ 28	$ 28	
Super Shine Marble Cleaner	N/A	1	$ 39	$ 39	
Dust Mop Treatment	BRA2080	1	$ 34	$ 34	
C-Fold Towel	FTJ244	5	$ 28	$ 138	
Toilet Paper	FTJ198	5	$ 45	$ 225	
Glass Cleaner	JAN7084	3	$ 43	$ 130	
Dust Mop Spray	BRA2080	2	$ 39	$ 78	
Giant Cleaner	DRK91218	2	$ 28	$ 56	
Facial Tissue	WIN920	3	$ 20	$ 59	
Trash Bag	JAGG4347G	2	$ 25	$ 50	
Clear Trash Bag	JAGL2432L	2	$ 25	$ 50	
Yellow Dust Cloth	FTJ296-16	2	$ 69	$ 138	
Pledge Lemon	DRK94399	2	$ 35	$ 70	
Dust Mop Frame	LBI1260	1	$ 10	$ 10	
Clip on Dust Mop Handle	LBI1490	1	$ 9	$ 9	
Industrial Dust Heads	LBI1060	2	$ 15	$ 30	
Stainless Steel Polish & Cleaner	SSI	2	$ 68	$ 136	
Tissue Box Covers	D9X-B8397	14	$ 27	$ 378	
Antislip Safety Strips	P6U-41008CL	8	$ 3	$ 22	
Q-tip holder	A58-1227	4	$ 7	$ 30	
Step Stools	S9R-1001-BLK	2	$ 55	$ 110	
Shaving gel		3	$ 36	$ 107	
Tampax	p/n HOS TAMPAX	1	$ 63	$ 63	
Urinal Blocks	p/n KRY UO3	2	$ 7	$ 14	
#566 Euro Platform ladder	p/n DAD ASPL5664	1	$ 65	$ 65	
8" Standard Trigger Sprayer/Bottles	p/n LAG5910-8	2	$ 2	$ 4	
Tampax Guards		1	$ 35	$ 35	
case of Eucalyptus fragrance		1	$ 130	$ 130	
R5U-9764 Door Wedge		10	$ 1	$ 13	
S5R-3559-GRY, 50 gallon refuse container		2	$ 78	$ 156	
disposable shower caps		5	$ 69	$ 345	
Shampoo (one 30 gallon drum)		1	$ 282	$ 282	
Conditioner (one 30 gallon drum)		1	$ 282	$ 282	
Antimicrobial Soap (one 30 gallon drum)		1	$ 289	$ 289	
Unscented Moisturizing Lotion (one 30 gallon drum)		1	$ 289	$ 289	
Morning Meadow Body Wash (one 30 gallon drum)		1	$ 289	$ 289	
Drum Pump (stainless steal and plastic)		2	$ 48	$ 95	
Morning Meadow Body Wash (gallons)		24	$ 13	$ 322	
Antimicrobial Soap (gallons)		8	$ 12	$ 93	
Gards feminine pads		1	$ 35	$ 35	
Garbage bags (50 gallon)		3	$ 25	$ 75	
facial tissue win 920		5	$ 20	$ 98	
triggers for spray bottles (8" standard for 24 oz. Bottles		8	$ 2	$ 16	
garbage can wheels-rcp-2610 gray				$ 100	
Sub-Total					$ 9,708
Sub-Total					$ 14,475
NJ Sales Tax @ 6%					$ 868
Freight & Installation @ 8%					$ 1,158
Contingency @ 2%					$ 289
Total					$ 16,791

Locker amenities and supplies.

Item - Client Linens		Unit Cost	Quantity	Cost
			Doz	
Hand Towels- Penthouse	16"x30"/Colonial Blue	$ 20	140	$ 2,800
Bath Towels- Penthouse	27"x54"/Colonial Blue	$ 69	140	$ 9,660
Sub-Total				$ 12,460
NJ Sales Tax @ 6%				$ 748
Freight & Installation @ 2.2%				$ 280
Total				$ 13,488

Member towels.

Rent Security	$ 65,625

Rent security.

Uniforms - Staff Assumptions			$ 100	Per Staff Per Yr Includes Tax & Shipping
Estimate $125 per staff member per year				
Yr 1 = 15				
Year	Staff/Yr	Annual Cost		
1	22	$ 2,200		
Sub-Total		$ 2,200		
NJ Sales Tax @ 6%		Included		
Freight & Installation @ 8%		Included		
Total		$ 2,200		

Staff uniforms.

X. FINANCIAL INFORMATION — SAMPLE 5-YEAR OPERATING BUDGET

	Dec-10	Jan-11	Feb-11	Mar-11	Apr-11	May-11	Jun-11	Jul-11	Aug-11	Sep-11	Oct-11	Nov-11	Dec-11	FYE 12.31.11
OPERATIONAL EXPENSES														
Rent	-	3,000	3,000	3,000	3,000	3,000	3,000	3,000	3,000	3,000	3,000	3,000	3,000	36,000
Marketing	-	2,160	2,160	2,160	2,160	2,160	2,160	2,160	2,160	2,160	2,160	2,160	2,160	25,915
Office Supplies	-	50	75	200	100	100	200	100		250	150	150	200	1,675
Uniforms	-	150			150			150	150		150			600
Water / Fruit	-													
Postage	-	3	5	2,107	9	12	14	16	2,167	20	22	24	26	4,426
Cable / Internet / Telephone	-	200	200	200	200	200	200	200	200	200	200	200	200	2,400
Biz Insurance	-	350	350	350	350	350	350	350	350	350	350	350	350	4,200
Insurance - GL&U	-	338	338	338	338	338	338	338	338	338	338	338	338	4,051
Insurance - Workers Comp	-	150	150	150	150	150	150	150	150	150	150	150	150	1,800
Maintenance / laundry	-													
Insurance	-													
Banking / Credit Card fees	-	262	321	380	438	512	559	617	676	747	806	865	924	7,106
Debt Service ($108,367 5 yr @ 9%)	-	2,250	2,250	2,250	2,250	2,250	2,250	2,250	2,250	2,250	2,250	2,250	2,250	27,000
	-	8,762	8,998	11,134	9,145	9,070	9,219	9,180	11,541	9,464	9,575	9,486	9,597	115,172
DIRECT EXPENSES														
Mgr's salary (75,000)	6,250	6,250	6,250	6,250	6,250	6,250	6,250	6,250	6,250	6,250	6,250	6,250	6,250	75,000
Payroll taxes (7,500)		625	625	625	625	625	625	625	625	625	625	625	625	7,500
Health Benefits (9,000)		750	750	750	750	750	750	750	750	750	750	750	750	9,000
Professional Dues / Travel				524					1,500		1,500			3,524
Trainers' pay			1,766	2,472	4,259	5,205	6,152	7,098	9,005	10,065	11,866	12,996	14,126	85,010
Trainers' p/r taxes			177	247	426	521	615	710	901	1,006	1,187	1,300	1,413	8,501
Benefits						521	615	710	901	1,006	1,187	1,300	1,413	7,651
Group Instructor's pay		1,400	1,400	1,400	1,400	1,400	800	800	800	1,400	1,400	1,400	1,400	15,000
Trainers' p/r taxes		140	140	140	140	140	80	80	80	140	140	140	140	1,500
Benefits														
	6,250	9,165	11,107	12,408	13,850	15,412	15,887	17,023	20,811	21,243	24,904	24,760	26,116	212,687
TOTAL EXPENSES	6,250	17,927	20,106	23,542	22,995	24,482	25,107	26,203	32,352	30,707	34,479	34,246	35,713	327,859
INCOME — staff trainers / sess/wk														
PT Revenue ($1695/24 sessions)		4,238	7,063	9,888	12,713	15,539	18,364	21,189	24,014	26,839	29,665	32,490	35,315	237,317
Ave #/wkly client-hrs		15	25	35	45	55	65	75	85	95	105	115	125	
# of client-hours		60	100	140	180	220	260	300	340	380	420	460	500	
$ per session		70.63	70.63	70.63	70.63	70.63	70.63	70.63	70.63	70.63	70.63	70.63	70.63	
Bootcamps Revenue		3,456	3,456	3,456	3,456	3,456	2,880	2,880	2,880	3,456	3,456	3,456	3,456	39,744
Ave #/classes per week		9	9	9	9	9	6	6	6	9	9	9	9	
Ave #/clients per class		8	8	8	8	8	10	10	10	8	8	8	8	
Ave #/wkly client-hrs		72	72	72	72	72	60	60	60	72	72	72	72	
# of clients-hours		288	288	288	288	288	240	240	240	288	288	288	288	
$ per client-hour (80%/$150/10 sessions)		12.00	12.00	12.00	12.00	12.00	12.00	12.00	12.00	12.00	12.00	12.00	12.00	
insPIRE Baseball Conditioning Revenue		3,446	3,446	3,446	3,446	4,136	4,136	4,136	4,136	4,136	4,136	4,136	4,136	46,871
Ave #/classes per week		8	8	8	8	8	8	8	8	8	8	8	8	
Ave #/clients per class		5	5	5	5	6	6	6	6	6	6	6	6	
Ave #/wkly client-hrs		40	40	40	40	48	48	48	48	48	48	48	48	
# of clients-hours		160	160	160	160	192	192	192	192	192	192	192	192	
$ per client-hour (80%/$350/13 sessions)		21.54	21.54	21.54	21.54	21.54	21.54	21.54	21.54	21.54	21.54	21.54	21.54	
TOTAL INCOME	-	11,140	13,965	16,791	19,616	23,130	25,379	28,205	31,030	34,431	37,256	40,081	42,907	323,932
EBITDA =	(6,250)	(6,787)	(6,140)	(6,752)	(3,379)	(1,352)	273	2,001	(1,322)	3,724	2,777	5,835	7,194	(3,927)
Accumulated net =	(6,250.00)	(6,787.07)	(12,927.21)	(19,679.01)	(23,058.17)	(24,409.78)	(24,136.85)	(22,135.39)	(23,457.65)	(19,733.41)	(16,956.18)	(11,120.77)	(3,927.21)	

Sports Training Academy Operating budget, year 1.

OPERATIONAL EXPENSES

	Dec-11	Jan-12	Feb-12	Mar-12	Apr-12	May-12	Jun-12	Jul-12	Aug-12	Sep-12	Oct-12	Nov-12	Dec-12	FYE 12.31.12
Rent	3,000	3,000	3,000	3,000	3,000	3,000	3,000	3,000	3,000	3,000	3,000	3,000	3,000	36,000
Marketing	2,160	4,156	4,156	4,156	4,156	4,156	4,156	4,156	4,156	4,156	4,156	4,156	4,156	49,967
Office Supplies	200	150	–	200	150	100	200	100	150	250	150	150	200	1,675
Uniforms	–	–	75	–	150	100	150	150	150	–	–	–	–	600
Water / fruit	–	–	–	–	–	–	–	–	–	–	–	–	–	–
Postage	26	27	28	2,129	30	32	33	34	2,184	36	37	38	39	4,646
Cable / Internet / Telephone	200	200	200	200	200	200	200	200	200	200	200	200	200	2,400
Biz Insurance	350	350	350	350	350	350	350	350	350	350	350	350	350	4,200
Insurance - GL&U	338	338	338	338	338	338	338	338	338	338	338	338	338	4,051
Insurance - Workers Comp	150	150	150	150	150	150	150	150	150	150	150	150	150	1,800
Maintenance / laundry														
Insurance / laundry														
Banking / Credit Card fees	924	953	982	1,012	1,041	1,071	1,088	1,117	1,147	1,188	1,218	1,247	1,277	13,341
Debt Service ($108,367 5 yr @ 9%)	2,250	2,250	2,250	2,250	2,250	2,250	2,250	2,250	2,250	2,250	2,250	2,250	2,250	27,000
	9,597	11,623	11,529	13,784	11,765	11,645	11,914	11,694	14,024	11,917	11,848	11,878	11,959	145,580

DIRECT EXPENSES

	Dec-11	Jan-12	Feb-12	Mar-12	Apr-12	May-12	Jun-12	Jul-12	Aug-12	Sep-12	Oct-12	Nov-12	Dec-12	FYE 12.31.12
Mgr's salary ($95,000)	6,250	7,917	7,917	7,917	7,917	7,917	7,917	7,917	7,917	7,917	7,917	7,917	7,917	95,000
Payroll taxes ($9,500)	625	792	792	792	792	792	792	792	792	792	792	792	792	9,500
Health Benefits ($9,000)	750	750	750	750	750	750	750	750	750	750	750	750	750	9,000
Professional Dues / Travel	–	–	–	524	–	–	–	–	1,500	–	1,500	–	–	3,524
Trainer's pay	14,126	18,364	19,070	19,776	20,483	21,189	21,895	22,602	23,308	24,014	24,721	25,427	26,133	266,981
Trainers' p/r taxes	1,413	1,836	1,907	1,978	2,048	2,119	2,190	2,260	2,331	2,401	2,472	2,543	2,613	26,698
Benefits	1,413	1,836	1,907	1,978	2,048	2,119	2,190	2,260	2,331	2,401	2,472	2,543	2,613	26,698
Group Instructor's pay	1,400	1,400	1,400	1,400	1,400	1,400	800	800	800	1,400	1,400	1,400	1,400	15,000
Trainers' p/r taxes	140	140	140	140	140	140	80	80	80	140	140	140	140	1,500
Benefits	140	140	140	140	140	140	80	80	80	140	140	140	140	1,500
	26,116	33,035	33,882	35,254	35,578	36,425	36,613	37,460	39,808	39,815	42,163	41,510	42,358	453,902
TOTAL EXPENSES	35,713	44,658	45,411	49,038	47,342	48,070	48,526	49,154	53,832	51,733	54,011	53,389	54,317	599,482

INCOME

	Dec-11	Jan-12	Feb-12	Mar-12	Apr-12	May-12	Jun-12	Jul-12	Aug-12	Sep-12	Oct-12	Nov-12	Dec-12	FYE 12.31.12
staff trainers	6	6	6	6	6	6	7	7	7	7	7	7	7	
sess/wk	22	22	23	23	24	25	22	23	24	24	25	26	26	
PT Revenue	35,315.00	36,728	38,140	39,553	40,965	42,378	43,791	45,203	46,616	48,028	49,441	50,854	52,266	533,963
Ave #/wkly client-hrs	125	130	135	140	145	150	155	160	165	170	175	180	185	
# of client-hours	500	520	540	560	580	600	620	640	660	680	700	720	740	
$ per session	70.63	70.63	70.63	70.63	70.63	70.63	70.63	70.63	70.63	70.63	70.63	70.63	70.63	
Bootcamps Revenue ($1695/24 sessions)	3,456.00	3,456	3,456	3,456	3,456	3,456	2,880	2,880	2,880	3,456	3,456	3,456	3,456	39,744
Ave #/classes per week	9	9	9	9	9	9	6	6	6	9	9	9	9	
Ave #/clients per class	8	8	8	8	8	8	10	10	10	8	8	8	8	
Ave #/wkly client-hrs (80%/$150/10 sessions)	72	72	72	72	72	72	60	60	60	72	72	72	72	
# of clients-hrs	288	288	288	288	288	288	240	240	240	288	288	288	288	
$ per client-hour	12.00	12.00	12.00	12.00	12.00	12.00	12.00	12.00	12.00	12.00	12.00	12.00	12.00	
insPIRE Baseball Conditioning Revenue	4,135.68	4,136	4,136	4,136	4,136	4,136	4,136	4,136	4,136	4,136	4,136	4,136	4,136	49,628
Ave #/classes per week	8.00	8	8	8	8	8	8	8	8	8	8	8	8	
Ave #/clients per class	6.00	6	6	6	6	6	6	6	6	6	6	6	6	
Ave #/wkly client-hrs	48.00	48	48	48	48	48	48	48	48	48	48	48	48	
# of clients-hours (80%/$350/13 sessions)	192.00	192	192	192	192	192	192	192	192	192	192	192	192	
$ per client-hour	21.54	21.54	21.54	21.54	21.54	21.54	21.54	21.54	21.54	21.54	21.54	21.54	21.54	
TOTAL INCOME	42,906.68	44,319	45,732	47,144	48,557	49,970	50,806	52,219	53,631	55,620	57,033	58,445	59,858	623,335
EBITDA =	7,193.57	(339)	321	(1,894)	1,215	1,899	2,280	3,064	(200)	3,888	3,022	5,057	5,541	23,853
Accumulated net =	(3,927.21)	(4,266.22)	(3,945.66)	(5,839.52)	(4,624.82)	(2,725.54)	(445.69)	2,618.73	2,418.54	6,306.11	9,328.25	14,384.97	19,926.25	

Sports Training Academy Operating budget, year 2.

OPERATIONAL EXPENSES

Item	Dec-12	Jan-13	Feb-13	Mar-13	Apr-13	May-13	Jun-13	Jul-13	Aug-13	Sep-13	Oct-13	Nov-13	Dec-13	FYE 12.31.13
Rent	3,000	3,000	3,000	3,000	3,000	3,000	3,000	3,000	3,000	3,000	3,000	3,000	3,000	36,000
Marketing	4,156	4,777	4,777	4,777	4,777	4,777	4,777	4,777	4,777	4,777	4,777	4,777	4,777	57,325
Office Supplies	200	1,675	75	200	100	100	200	100	100	250	150	150	200	3,300
Uniforms	-	600	-	-	150	-	-	-	150	-	-	-	-	900
Water / fruit	-	-	-	-	-	-	-	-	-	-	-	-	-	-
Postage	39	39	39	2,139	39	39	39	39	2,188	39	39	39	39	4,715
Cable / Internet / Telephone	200	200	200	200	200	200	200	200	200	200	200	200	200	2,400
Biz Insurance	350	350	350	350	350	350	350	350	350	350	350	350	350	4,200
Insurance - GL&U	338	338	338	338	338	338	338	338	338	338	338	338	338	4,051
Insurance - Workers Comp	150	150	150	150	150	150	150	150	150	150	150	150	150	1,800
Maintenance / laundry														
Insurance														
Banking / Credit Card fees	1,277	1,277	1,277	1,277	1,277	1,277	1,265	1,265	1,265	1,277	1,277	1,277	1,277	15,282
Debt Service	2,250	2,250	2,250	2,250	2,250	2,250	2,250	2,250	2,250	2,250	2,250	2,250	2,250	27,000
Operating total	11,959	14,655	12,455	14,680	12,630	12,480	12,568	12,468	14,767	12,630	12,530	12,530	12,580	156,974

Debt Service annotation: $108,367 5 yr @ 9%

DIRECT EXPENSES

Item	Dec-12	Jan-13	Feb-13	Mar-13	Apr-13	May-13	Jun-13	Jul-13	Aug-13	Sep-13	Oct-13	Nov-13	Dec-13	FYE 12.31.13
Mgr's salary	7,917	10,417	10,417	10,417	10,417	10,417	10,417	10,417	10,417	10,417	10,417	10,417	10,417	125,000
Payroll taxes	792	1,042	1,042	1,042	1,042	1,042	1,042	1,042	1,042	1,042	1,042	1,042	1,042	12,500
Health Benefits	750	750	750	750	750	750	750	750	750	750	750	750	750	9,000
Professional Dues / Travel	-	-	-	524	-	-	-	-	1,500	-	1,500	-	-	3,524
Trainer's pay	26,133	26,133	26,133	26,133	26,133	26,133	26,133	26,133	26,133	26,133	26,133	26,133	26,133	313,597
Trainers' p/r taxes	2,613	2,613	2,613	2,613	2,613	2,613	2,613	2,613	2,613	2,613	2,613	2,613	2,613	31,360
Benefits	2,613	2,613	2,613	2,613	2,613	2,613	2,613	2,613	2,613	2,613	2,613	2,613	2,613	31,360
Group Instructor's pay	1,400	1,400	1,400	1,400	1,400	1,400	800	800	800	1,400	1,400	1,400	1,400	15,000
Trainers' p/r taxes	140	140	140	140	140	140	80	80	80	140	140	140	140	1,500
Benefits	140	140	140	140	140	140	80	80	80	140	140	140	140	1,500
Direct total	42,358	45,108	45,108	45,632	45,108	45,108	44,448	44,448	45,948	45,108	46,608	45,108	45,108	542,841

Mgr's salary box: $125,000 — Payroll taxes box: $12,500 — Health Benefits box: $9,000

	Dec-12	Jan-13	Feb-13	Mar-13	Apr-13	May-13	Jun-13	Jul-13	Aug-13	Sep-13	Oct-13	Nov-13	Dec-13	FYE 12.31.13
TOTAL EXPENSES	54,317	59,763	57,563	60,312	57,738	57,588	57,016	56,916	60,715	57,738	59,138	57,638	57,688	699,815

INCOME

Item	Dec-12	Jan-13	Feb-13	Mar-13	Apr-13	May-13	Jun-13	Jul-13	Aug-13	Sep-13	Oct-13	Nov-13	Dec-13	FYE 12.31.13
PT Revenue	52,266.20	52,266	52,266	52,266	52,266	52,266	52,266	52,266	52,266	52,266	52,266	52,266	52,266	627,194
staff trainers	7	7	7	7	7	7	7	7	7	7	7	7	7	
sess/wk	26	26	26	26	26	26	26	26	26	26	26	26	26	
Ave #wkly client-hrs	185	185	185	185	185	185	185	185	185	185	185	185	185	
# of client-hours	740	740	740	740	740	740	740	740	740	740	740	740	740	
$ per session	70.63	70.63	70.63	70.63	70.63	70.63	70.63	70.63	70.63	70.63	70.63	70.63	70.63	
Bootcamps Revenue	3,456.00	3,456	3,456	3,456	3,456	3,456	2,880	2,880	2,880	3,456	3,456	3,456	3,456	39,744
Ave #classes per week	9	8	8	8	8	8	6	6	6	8	8	8	8	
Ave #clients per class	8	9	9	9	9	9	10	10	10	9	9	9	9	
Ave #wkly client-hrs	72	72	72	72	72	72	60	60	60	72	72	72	72	
# of clients-hours	288	288	288	288	288	288	240	240	240	288	288	288	288	
$ per client-hour	12.00	12.00	12.00	12.00	12.00	12.00	12.00	12.00	12.00	12.00	12.00	12.00	12.00	
insPIRE Baseball Conditioning Revenue	4,135.68	4,136	4,136	4,136	4,136	4,136	4,136	4,136	4,136	4,136	4,136	4,136	4,136	49,628
Ave #classes per week	8	8	8	8	8	8	8	8	8	8	8	8	8	
Ave #clients per class	6	6	6	6	6	6	6	6	6	6	6	6	6	
Ave #wkly client-hrs	48	48	48	48	48	48	48	48	48	48	48	48	48	
# of clients-hours	192	192	192	192	192	192	192	192	192	192	192	192	192	
$ per client-hour	21.54	21.54	21.54	21.54	21.54	21.54	21.54	21.54	21.54	21.54	21.54	21.54	21.54	

PT Revenue annotation: $1695/24 sessions — Bootcamps annotation: 80%/$150/10 sessions — insPIRE annotation: 80%/$350/13 sessions

	Dec-12	Jan-13	Feb-13	Mar-13	Apr-13	May-13	Jun-13	Jul-13	Aug-13	Sep-13	Oct-13	Nov-13	Dec-13	FYE 12.31.13
TOTAL INCOME	59,857.88	59,858	59,858	59,858	59,858	59,858	59,282	59,282	59,282	59,858	59,858	59,858	59,858	716,567
EBITDA =	5,541.29	95	2,295	(454)	2,120	2,270	2,266	2,366	(1,433)	2,120	720	2,220	2,170	16,752
Accumulated net =	19,926.25	20,020.99	22,315.74	21,861.48	23,981.22	26,250.97	28,516.70	30,882.44	29,449.10	31,568.85	32,288.59	34,508.33	36,678.07	

Sports Training Academy Operating budget, year 3.

OPERATIONAL EXPENSES

	Dec-13	Jan-14	Feb-14	Mar-14	Apr-14	May-14	Jun-14	Jul-14	Aug-14	Sep-14	Oct-14	Nov-14	Dec-14	FYE 12.31.14
Rent	3,000	3,000	3,000	3,000	3,000	3,000	3,000	3,000	3,000	3,000	3,000	3,000	3,000	36,000
Marketing	4,156	4,777	4,777	4,777	4,777	4,777	4,777	4,777	4,777	4,777	4,777	4,777	4,777	57,325
Office Supplies	200	1,675	75	200	100	100	200	100	100	250	150	150	200	3,300
Uniforms		600			150				150					900
Water / fruit														
Postage	39	39	39	2,139	39	39	39	39	2,188	39	39	39	39	4,715
Cable / Internet / Telephone	200	200	200	200	200	200	200	200	200	200	200	200	200	2,400
Biz Insurance	350	350	350	350	350	350	350	350	350	350	350	350	350	4,200
Insurance - GL&U	338	338	338	338	338	338	338	338	338	338	338	338	338	4,051
Insurance - Workers Comp	150	150	150	150	150	150	150	150	150	150	150	150	150	1,800
Maintenance / laundry														
Insurance														
Insurance Plan														
Banking / Credit Card fees	1,277	1,277	1,277	1,277	1,277	1,277	1,265	1,265	1,265	1,277	1,277	1,277	1,277	15,282
Debt Service	2,250	2,250	2,250	2,250	2,250	2,250	2,250	2,250	2,250	2,250	2,250	2,250	2,250	27,000
	11,959	14,655	12,455	14,680	12,630	12,480	12,568	12,468	14,767	12,630	12,530	12,530	12,580	156,974

$108,367 5 yr @ 9%

DIRECT EXPENSES

	Dec-13	Jan-14	Feb-14	Mar-14	Apr-14	May-14	Jun-14	Jul-14	Aug-14	Sep-14	Oct-14	Nov-14	Dec-14	FYE 12.31.14
Mgr's salary	10,417	10,417	10,417	10,417	10,417	10,417	10,417	10,417	10,417	10,417	10,417	10,417	10,417	125,000
Payroll taxes	1,042	1,042	1,042	1,042	1,042	1,042	1,042	1,042	1,042	1,042	1,042	1,042	1,042	12,500
Health Benefits	750	750	750	750	750	750	750	750	750	750	750	750	750	9,000
Professional Dues / Travel				524					1,500		1,500			3,524
Trainer's pay	26,133	26,133	26,133	26,133	26,133	26,133	26,133	26,133	26,133	26,133	26,133	26,133	26,133	313,597
Trainers' p/r taxes	2,613	2,613	2,613	2,613	2,613	2,613	2,613	2,613	2,613	2,613	2,613	2,613	2,613	31,360
Benefits	2,613	2,613	2,613	2,613	2,613	2,613	2,613	2,613	2,613	2,613	2,613	2,613	2,613	31,360
Group Instructor's pay	1,400	1,400	1,400	1,400	1,400	1,400	800	800	800	1,400	1,400	1,400	1,400	15,000
Trainers' p/r taxes	140	140	140	140	140	140	80	80	80	140	140	140	140	1,500
Benefits														
	45,108	45,108	45,108	45,632	45,108	45,108	44,448	44,448	45,948	45,108	46,608	45,108	45,108	542,841

(annual: 125,000 / 12,500 / 9,000)

	Dec-13	Jan-14	Feb-14	Mar-14	Apr-14	May-14	Jun-14	Jul-14	Aug-14	Sep-14	Oct-14	Nov-14	Dec-14	FYE 12.31.14
TOTAL EXPENSES	57,067	59,763	57,563	60,312	57,738	57,588	57,016	56,916	60,715	57,738	59,138	57,638	57,688	699,815

INCOME

	Dec-13	Jan-14	Feb-14	Mar-14	Apr-14	May-14	Jun-14	Jul-14	Aug-14	Sep-14	Oct-14	Nov-14	Dec-14	FYE 12.31.14
staff trainers	7	7	7	7	7	7	7	7	7	7	7	7	7	
sess/wk	26	26	26	26	26	26	26	26	26	26	26	26	26	
PT Revenue	52,266.20	52,266	52,266	52,266	52,266	52,266	52,266	52,266	52,266	52,266	52,266	52,266	52,266	627,194
Ave #/wkly client-hrs	185.00	185	185	185	185	185	185	185	185	185	185	185	185	
# of client-hours	740.00	740	740	740	740	740	740	740	740	740	740	740	740	
$1695/24 sessions $ per session	70.63	70.63	70.63	70.63	70.63	70.63	70.63	70.63	70.63	70.63	70.63	70.63	70.63	
Bootcamps Revenue	3,456.00	3,456	3,456	3,456	3,456	3,456	2,880	2,880	2,880	3,456	3,456	3,456	3,456	39,744
Ave #/classes per week	9.00	9	9	9	9	9	6	6	6	9	9	9	9	
Ave #/clients per class	8.00	8	8	8	8	8	10	10	10	8	8	8	8	
Ave #/wkly client-hrs	72.00	72	72	72	72	72	60	60	60	72	72	72	72	
# of clients-hours	288.00	288	288	288	288	288	240	240	240	288	288	288	288	
80%/$150/10 sessions $ per client-hour	12.00	12.00	12.00	12.00	12.00	12.00	12.00	12.00	12.00	12.00	12.00	12.00	12.00	
insPIRE Baseball Conditioning Revenue	4,135.68	4,136	4,136	4,136	4,136	4,136	4,136	4,136	4,136	4,136	4,136	4,136	4,136	49,628
Ave #/classes per week	8.00	8	8	8	8	8	8	8	8	8	8	8	8	
Ave #/clients per class	6.00	6	6	6	6	6	6	6	6	6	6	6	6	
Ave #/wkly client-hrs	48.00	48	48	48	48	48	48	48	48	48	48	48	48	
# of clients-hours	192.00	192	192	192	192	192	192	192	192	192	192	192	192	
80%/$350/13 sessions $ per client-hour	21.54	21.54	21.54	21.54	21.54	21.54	21.54	21.54	21.54	21.54	21.54	21.54	21.54	
TOTAL INCOME	59,857.88	59,858	59,858	59,858	59,858	59,858	59,282	59,282	59,282	59,858	59,858	59,858	59,858	716,567
EBITDA =	2,169.74	95	2,295	(454)	2,120	2,270	2,266	2,366	(1,433)	2,120	720	2,220	2,170	16,752
Accumulated net =	36,678.07	36,772.82	39,067.56	38,613.30	40,733.04	43,002.79	45,268.52	47,634.26	46,200.93	48,320.67	49,040.41	51,260.15	53,429.90	

Sports Training Academy Operating budget, year 4.

OPERATIONAL EXPENSES

	Dec-14	Jan-15	Feb-15	Mar-15	Apr-15	May-15	Jun-15	Jul-15	Aug-15	Sep-15	Oct-15	Nov-15	Dec-15	FYE 12.31.15
Rent	3,000	3,000	3,000	3,000	3,000	3,000	3,000	3,000	3,000	3,000	3,000	3,000	3,000	36,000
Marketing	4,777	4,777	4,777	4,777	4,777	4,777	4,777	4,777	4,777	4,777	4,777	4,777	4,777	57,325
Office Supplies	200	1,675	75	200	100	100	200	100	100	250	150	150	200	3,300
Uniforms		600			150				150					900
Water / fruit														
Postage	39	39	39	2,139	39	39	39	39	2,188	39	39	39	39	4,715
Cable / Internet / Telephone	200	200	200	200	200	200	200	200	200	200	200	200	200	2,400
Biz Insurance	350	350	350	350	350	350	350	350	350	350	350	350	350	4,200
Insurance - GL&U	338	338	338	338	338	338	338	338	338	338	338	338	338	4,051
Insurance - Workers Comp	150	150	150	150	150	150	150	150	150	150	150	150	150	1,800
Maintenance / laundry														
Insurance														
Banking / Credit Card fees	1,277	1,277	1,277	1,277	1,277	1,277	1,265	1,265	1,265	1,277	1,277	1,277	1,277	15,282
Debt Service	2,250	2,250	2,250	2,250	2,250	2,250	2,250	2,250	2,250	2,250	2,250	2,250	2,250	27,000
	12,580	14,655	12,455	14,680	12,630	12,480	12,568	12,468	14,767	12,630	12,530	12,530	12,580	156,974

$108,367 5 yr @ 9% (Debt Service)

DIRECT EXPENSES

	Dec-14	Jan-15	Feb-15	Mar-15	Apr-15	May-15	Jun-15	Jul-15	Aug-15	Sep-15	Oct-15	Nov-15	Dec-15	FYE 12.31.15
Mgr's salary	10,417	10,417	10,417	10,417	10,417	10,417	10,417	10,417	10,417	10,417	10,417	10,417	10,417	125,000
Payroll taxes	1,042	1,042	1,042	1,042	1,042	1,042	1,042	1,042	1,042	1,042	1,042	1,042	1,042	12,500
Health Benefits	750	750	750	750	750	750	750	750	750	750	750	750	750	9,000
Professional Dues / Travel				524					1,500		1,500			3,524
Trainer's pay	26,133	26,133	26,133	26,133	26,133	26,133	26,133	26,133	26,133	26,133	26,133	26,133	26,133	313,597
Trainers' p/r taxes	2,613	2,613	2,613	2,613	2,613	2,613	2,613	2,613	2,613	2,613	2,613	2,613	2,613	31,360
Benefits	2,613	2,613	2,613	2,613	2,613	2,613	2,613	2,613	2,613	2,613	2,613	2,613	2,613	31,360
Group Instructor's pay	1,400	1,400	1,400	1,400	1,400	1,400	800	800	800	1,400	1,400	1,400	1,400	15,000
Trainers' p/r taxes	140	140	140	140	140	140	80	80	80	140	140	140	140	1,500
Benefits	140	140	140	140	140	140	80	80	80	140	140	140	140	1,500
	45,108	45,108	45,108	45,632	45,108	45,108	44,448	44,448	45,948	45,108	46,608	45,108	45,108	542,841
TOTAL EXPENSES	57,688	59,763	57,563	60,312	57,738	57,588	57,016	56,916	60,715	57,738	59,138	57,638	57,688	699,815

125,000 / 12,500 / 9,000

INCOME (staff trainers / sess/wk)

	Dec-14	Jan-15	Feb-15	Mar-15	Apr-15	May-15	Jun-15	Jul-15	Aug-15	Sep-15	Oct-15	Nov-15	Dec-15	FYE 12.31.15
PT Revenue	52,266.20	52,266	52,266	52,266	52,266	52,266	52,266	52,266	52,266	52,266	52,266	52,266	52,266	627,194
Ave #/wkly client-hrs	185.00	185	185	185	185	185	185	185	185	185	185	185	185	
# of client-hours	740.00	740	740	740	740	740	740	740	740	740	740	740	740	
$ per session	70.63	70.63	70.63	70.63	70.63	70.63	70.63	70.63	70.63	70.63	70.63	70.63	70.63	
Bootcamps Revenue	3,456.00	3,456	3,456	3,456	3,456	3,456	2,880	2,880	2,880	3,456	3,456	3,456	3,456	39,744
Ave #/classes per week	9.00	9	9	9	9	9	6	6	6	9	9	9	9	
Ave #/clients per class	8.00	8	8	8	8	8	10	10	10	8	8	8	8	
Ave #/wkly client-hrs	72.00	72	72	72	72	72	60	60	60	72	72	72	72	
# of clients-hours	288.00	288	288	288	288	288	240	240	240	288	288	288	288	
$ per client-hour	12.00	12.00	12.00	12.00	12.00	12.00	12.00	12.00	12.00	12.00	12.00	12.00	12.00	
Baseball Conditioning Revenue	4,135.68	4,136	4,136	4,136	4,136	4,136	4,136	4,136	4,136	4,136	4,136	4,136	4,136	49,628
Ave #/classes per week	8.00	8	8	8	8	8	8	8	8	8	8	8	8	
Ave #/clients per class	6.00	6	6	6	6	6	6	6	6	6	6	6	6	
Ave #/wkly client-hrs	48.00	48	48	48	48	48	48	48	48	48	48	48	48	
# of clients-hours	192.00	192	192	192	192	192	192	192	192	192	192	192	192	
$ per client-hour	21.54	21.54	21.54	21.54	21.54	21.54	21.54	21.54	21.54	21.54	21.54	21.54	21.54	
TOTAL INCOME	59,857.88	59,858	59,858	59,858	59,858	59,858	59,282	59,282	59,282	59,858	59,858	59,858	59,858	716,567
EBITDA =	2,169.74	95	2,295	(454)	2,120	2,270	2,266	2,366	(1,433)	2,120	720	2,220	2,170	16,752
Accumulated net =	53,429.90	53,524.64	55,819.38	55,365.12	57,484.87	59,754.61	62,020.35	64,386.08	62,952.75	65,072.49	65,792.23	68,011.97	70,181.72	70,181.72

$1695/24 sessions (PT Revenue / Bootcamps Revenue)
80%/$150/10 sessions (Bootcamps)
insPIRE Baseball Conditioning Revenue
80%/$350/13 sessions (Baseball Conditioning)

Sports Training Academy Operating budget, year 5.

Triad Fitness

- Adult Fitness
- Sports Training Academy
- Youth Fitness Zone

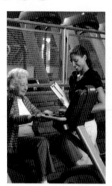

Surgeon General's Report: Benefits of Fitness for "All Generations"

Reduction of Coronary Risk Factors

- Reduction of total cholesterol
  - Improvement of HDL
  - Reduction of LDL
  - Reduction of triglycerides
- Improvement of body composition
- Lowering of blood pressure
- Lowering of resting heart rate

Overview of Triad Fitness

- Premium provider of ***MEDICALLY ORIENTED PROGRAMS***
  - Adults
  - Children
  - Sports training programs
- Location: Allendale, NJ
  - Population: 167,500 in an 8 mile radius
  - Mean family income: $153,000

Overview of Triad Fitness

- Size of Facility: 17,500 Square Feet
  - Adult program: 10,000 sq. ft.
  - Sports Training Academy & Youth Fitness Zone: 7,500 sq. ft.

Adult Fitness Program

Adult Physical Fitness

Primary Target Market

- Mature (35+), affluent, well educated, physically deconditioned, men and women
- Want to take an active role in their preventive health care
- Average household income: $120,000
- There are no firms within the demographic target market that deliver ***medically oriented programs***

Adult Physical Fitness

Typical Membership Program

■Fees
- Membership fees: $960/ year OR $80/ month
- Assessment Fee: $99 one time charge

■Entry Procedures
- PARQ (Physical Activity Readiness Questionnaire)
- Medical History Form from personal MD (if required)
- Physical Fitness Assessment
- Individual Program Implementation

Adult Physical Fitness

Typical Membership Program (cont'd)

■ Exercise Programming
- Reassessment after 9-10 months
- Group exercise classes

Additional Services

■ Personal Training
- 12 Sessions: $780 or $65/session
- 24 Sessions: $1,440 or $60/session

Children's Programs

Youth Fitness Zone
Sports Training Academy

Children's Programs Overview

Primary Target Market
- Family Income of $75,000 or more
- Age range: 8-20 years old
- Market segmentation: 15 mile radius from Allendale, NJ
- 300,000 Children within a 15 mile radius

Youth Fitness Zone

Youth Fitness Zone (YFZ)

Child Obesity (CDC 2000)

- 15% of the population of children are either overweight or obese
- Another 15% are designated "at risk"
- Surgeon General's Call to Action 2001
  - Reduce TV Watching
  - Promote healthier food choices
  - 60 minutes of moderate daily activity most days of the week

Youth Fitness Zone (YFZ)

Child Obesity (cont'd)

- Public schools' physical education programs are falling short.
- Parents of these children would like to help:
  - improve their Child's self-esteem
  - improve their Child's health
  - improve their Child's sense of camaraderie with their peers.

Youth Fitness Zone (YFZ)

Typical Youth Fitness Zone Program

- There are no firms within the demographic target market that deliver *medically oriented programs*
  - Health History Questionnaire
  - Medical History Form from personal MD (if required)
  - Physical Fitness Assessment
  - Program Implementation

Youth Fitness Zone

Program Fees

- Assessment: $95
- Group Training:
  - 12 Sessions: $295 or $24.58/session
  - 24 Sessions: $575 or $23.96/session
- Personal Training: $60/ session

Sports Training Academy

Sports Training Academy (STA)

Current Market

- Recreational and interscholastic athletics are becoming increasingly competitive
  - Parents want to give their children the "competitive edge" in order to be "on top of their game"
- American households with children spent an estimated $4.1 billion last year on sports instruction and private coaching

Sports Training Academy

Typical STA Program

- Health History Questionnaire
- Medical History Form from personal MD (if required)
- Physical Performance Assessment
  - If appropriate a referral is made to Youth Fitness Zone in order to increase levels of physical fitness

Sports Training Academy

Typical STA Program (cont'd)

- Program Implementation of Training Protocols
  - Scientifically designed to maximize "individual" athletic potential & sport(s) performance

Program Fees

- Assessment: $95
- Group Training
  - 12 Sessions: $360 or $30.00/session
  - 24 Sessions: $695 or $28.95/session

Sports Training Academy

- Parents – Just Like every parent, you want the best for your child.
- Coaches – For your athletes, performance is everything.
- Students – Now is the time to achieve your dreams.

Marketing and Advertising

Marketing & Advertising Strategy

- Experienced advertising agency will be retained
- Build "brand" awareness
- Differentiate Triad Fitness services and programs from your "typical health club" market
  - Professional staff
  - Medically oriented programs
  - Limited membership capacity
  - 30-Day Guarantee

Marketing & Advertising Strategy (cont'd)

- Aggressive, targeted advertising and marketing with a budget of $106,100 for the first year
- There are no firms within the demographic target market that deliver ***medically oriented programs,*** which our strategy will take in account

Why 3 Programs Under One Roof?

- The 3 programs under the same roof create a very effective cross-referral system
- Kids do not drive!!
  - After driving their kids to regular visits at the facility, many parents enroll as adult fitness members
  - Many parents who don't enroll, visit the juice bar while waiting for their children
  - Adult fitness members see the children's program first-hand and enroll their kids in the Youth Fitness Zone and/or STA program

Financials

5 Year EBITDA*

	Year 1	Year 2	Year 3	Year 4	Year 5
Total Revenue	$ 1,526,889	$ 2,746,531	$ 5,525,079	$ 8,906,555	$ 13,332,866
Total Direct Expenses	$ 950,304	$ 1,401,351	$ 2,530,707	$ 3,756,047	$5,386,168
Total Operating Expenses	$ 535,132	$ 686,242	$ 1,362,488	$ 2,119,180	$ 2,988,453
Operating Profit	**$41,453**	**$ 658,938**	**$ 1,631,884**	**$ 3,031,329**	**$ 4,958,245**
Bonus	$ 0	$ 65,894	$ 152,583	$ 283,016	$ 473,818
Benefits	$ 0	$ 16,473	$ 38,146	$ 70,754	$ 118,455
EBITDA	**$ 41,453**	**$ 576,571**	**$ 1,441,155**	**$ 2,677,599**	**$ 4,365,972**
% of Revenue	**2.71%**	**20.99%**	**26.08%**	**30.06%**	**32.75%**

* 5 year analysis with 1 New Center going on line each year starting in Year 3

5 Year Consolidated Statement of Earnings*

	Year 1	Year 2	Year 3	Year 4	Year 5
Revenue					
Adult	$ 620,840	$ 1,410,788	$ 2, 808,897	$ 4,633,003	$ 7,029,542
STA	$ 457,200	$ 610,555	$ 1,254,770	$ 1,959,065	$ 2,830,138
YFZ	$ 303,420	$ 465,560	$ 946,220	$ 1,488,396	$ 2,209,656
Other**	$ 145,429	$ 259,628	$ 515,192	$ 826,091	$ 1,263,530
Total Revenue	**$ 1,526,889**	**$ 2,746,531**	**$ 5,525,079**	**$ 8,906,555**	**$ 13,332,866**
Total Direct Expense	**($ 950,304)**	**($ 1,401,351)**	**($ 2,530,707)**	**($ 3,756,047)**	**($ 5,386,168)**

*5 year analysis with 1 New Center going on line each year starting in Year 3
** Includes: nutritional services, child care programs, juice bar, athletic wear, camps

5 Year Consolidated Statement of Earnings

	Year 1	Year 2	Year 3	Year 4	Year 5
Operating Expenses					
Rent, CAM, Utilities	$ 213,775	$ 214,615	$ 439,630	$ 673,580	$ 909,457
Advertising & Promotions	$ 61,076	$ 109,861	$ 217,798	$ 344,855	$ 513,493
Other	$ 260,281	$ 361,765	$ 705,060	$ 1,100,745	$ 1,565,503
Total Operating Expenses	**($ 535,132)**	**($ 686,242)**	**($ 1,362,488)**	**($ 2,119,180)**	**($ 2,988,453)**

5 Year Consolidated Statement of Earnings

	Year 1	Year 2	Year 3	Year 4	Year 5
Operating Profit	$ 41,453	$ 658,938	$ 1,631,884	$ 3,031,329	$ 4,958,245
Bonus	0	($ 65,894)	($ 152,583)	($ 283,016)	($ 473,818)
Benefits	0	($ 16,473)	($ 38,146)	($ 70,754)	($ 118,455)
Depreciation (7 years)	($ 80,141)	($ 80,141)	($ 160,281)	($ 240,422)	($ 320,563)
Amortization (15 years)	($ 114,688)	($ 114,688)	($ 229,375)	($ 344,063)	($ 458,750)

5 Year Consolidated Statement of Earnings

	Year 1	Year 2	Year 3	Year 4	Year 5
Earnings Before Taxes	($ 153,375)	$ 381,743	$ 1,051,499	$ 2,093,074	$ 3,586,659
Corporate Taxes (35%)	0	($ 79,930)*	($ 368,025)	($ 732,576)	($ 1,255,331)
Net Earnings	($ 153,375)	$ 301,813	$ 683,474	$ 1,360,498	$ 2,331,328
% of Revenue	(10.00%)	10.99%	12.37%	15.28%	17.49%
Cumulative Net Earnings	($ 153,375)	$ 148,438	$ 831,912	$ 2,192,410	$ 4,523,738

*Includes Tax Loss Carry forward from prior year

Index

Page numbers in *italics* denote figures; those followed by b denote boxes.